INTERMITTENT FASTING FOR WOMEN OVER 50

The Complete Guide to Lose Weight, Detox Your Body and Improve Your Health With Intermittent Fasting

Dayna Andy

TABLE OF CONTENTS

INTRODUCTION

Congratulations on purchasing this book, and thank you for doing so. This book will help you in understanding the concept of intermittent fasting for women over 50.

Entering the 50s can be a revelation. Things begin to change rapidly. The most significant change comes on the health front. The small issues that you had been ignoring or brushing aside easily for the past, so many years all of a sudden emerge as real chronic illnesses. The things that you felt would improve automatically with menopause or vanish completely appear in a new and more vicious form.

Navigating the 50s can be a daunting task for many women in the beginning. It brings with itself a lot of health challenges for which you might not be fully prepared. Chronic illnesses can become a real headache in the 50s. It is also the time your immunity starts failing you.

There are many hormonal issues that most women face but are unable to figure out a way to deal with them. Obesity also emerges as a bigger problem as your tendency to gain weight increases all of a sudden.

The 50s can be the point where you come across many such issues and may not be able to understand the correct strategy to navigate easily.

Intermittent fasting is one of the best ways for women to find ways into good health in their 50s. It is easy to follow, effective, and very efficient way to stay healthy and fit.

Losing weight is the easiest with intermittent fasting, as it can help you in reaching ketosis fast. You will not only lose weight but will also be able to burn the adamant belly fat too.

Intermittent fasting is also a savior for women over 50, as it can help in initiating autophagy. This is the process that can bring amazing anti-aging properties and also heal your body from within. It can also help in eliminating long-standing allergies, immunity issues, and chronic inflammations.

This is a comprehensive book for women over 50 who want to understand intermittent fasting in detail. It would explain the health issues that you face and how intermittent fasting can help you in solving them.

It would not only present the tall claims but would also explain the functioning of intermittent fasting in a detailed manner.

From various intermittent fasting protocols specifically suitable for women over 50 to the ways through which initiating ketosis and autophagy will be easy, this book will cover everything in vivid detail.

This book has been written as a guide book for women over 50 so that they can find the solution for their health issues in this book easily.

Every claim in this book will have an explanation so that you can understand if that can work for you or not.

From tips and tricks to manage the side-effects to major dietary changes needed for better results, this book will throw light on every aspect of Intermittent Fasting.

This book has been written in a very simple and easy to understand way so that everyone can take advantage of this information.

I hope that you will be able to get the full advantage of this book.

There are plenty of books on this subject on the market, thanks again for choosing this one! Every effort was made to ensure it is full of as much useful information as possible; please enjoy it!

CHAPTER 1

IMPACT OF AGING ON OVERALL HEALTH OF WOMEN

Longevity- A Boon or a Curse for Women?

Life is a gift. We all want it to be very long or even eternal.

One of the most untiring pursuits of humankind has been to find secrets of immortality. We may not have been fully successful in that, yet we have found ways to lengthen the lifespan.

Despite the pollution, toxicity, chemicals, weapons of mass destruction, and all other such scary stuff, you'd appreciate the fact that the average human lifespan has increased considerably. If we just go back a little in the past, the average human lifespan has never been half of what it is today.

Today, the average life expectancy in the US is above 80 years. In the 1800s, the average life expectancy in most of the countries was well below 25 years. Belgium had the best life expectancy rates then, and even there the best estimate was 40 years.

Thankfully, modern medical science has made tremendous progress. At the beginning of the 20th Century, life expectancy in the US was less than 50 years. In just a century, at the beginning of the 21st Century, life expectancy in the US stands above 80 years.

Although long life is a boon and humanity along with modern medical science had been working very hard to achieve it, long life without youth and vigor is of little consequence. It is a fact that none of us would want to die early, and every person even on the death bed at the fag end of life, still struggles to catch the last breath.

Yet, a weak, painful, and dependent life is not exactly what people may have had on their minds when they must have started thinking about a long life.

Women are especially at the poor receiving end of this gift of long life.

Statistically speaking, women have an even better life expectancy rates than men and some worse problems than them.

Some Hard Facts

Straightaway, let us dig into some hard facts.

As I mentioned above, women have better life expectancy rates than men. Currently, in the US, men have a life expectancy of 76.1 years, while women live up to 81.1 years. That is a gap of 5 years. This is a gap that has been widening consistently over the years.

In the year 1900, the life expectancy in men was 46.3 while in women, it was 48.3. There was just a 2-year gap.

This may sound like a good thing, but in reality, it isn't. Aging doesn't come alone. It brings with itself a lot of health problems.

Aging is generally associated with weakening of muscles, declining eyesight, poor memory, limited mobility, and many other such problems.

This age gap also highlights the fact that women are more likely to outlive their partners, and that means living alone in a state in which they are more dependent and vulnerable.

Center for Disease Control and Prevention (CDC) fact sheet states that 43% of women above the age of 65 are likely to get widowed. The percentage of men likely to get widowed by this age is just 13%.

Not only this, but 38% of older women are also likely to live alone. This percentage for men is just 19%.

The reason for this difference is that women are more likely to live longer. They are more likely to outlive their partners.

This should have been a good thing from the longevity perspective, but because with longevity aging also come into the picture, this whole thing turns bad.

Till now, we have only been looking at the fact that women are more likely to live longer than men.

Women are also more likely to have chronic illnesses, and they will be forced to cope with these issues all by themselves at an age when their health would be failing rapidly.

Data suggests that although women are more likely to live longer, they are also more likely to get affected by a higher number of chronic illnesses, which can make their later part of life even more difficult.

For instance, between the age group of 65-74, around 67.4% of women are expected to be suffering from high blood pressure whereas this percentage is around 61.1% in men.

Likewise, 43.5% of women are expected to be obese by this age, while this percentage will only be 40.2% in men belonging to the same age group.

As per the National Health and Nutrition Examination Survey (NHANES) reports, around 33% of all women above 50 are likely to suffer from heart conditions. This percentage is 26% for the men of the same age group.

For arthritis, this percentage is 51% in women and 40% in men. The National Osteoporosis Foundation report suggests that more than 10 million Americans are currently suffering from Osteoporosis, and even in this 80% of the patients are women. It further goes on to say that at least one out of two women above the age of 50 will break a bone due to the problem. Not only this, but the risk of breaking a hip in women is also equal to the combined risk of break, uterine, and ovarian cancer.

Heart problems and diabetes are some of the most common chronic illnesses people face these days. Both these problems are the cause of the highest number of deaths in the US. Although these diseases are fatal enough in themselves, if a person suffers from both the risk increases manifolds.

Data states that around 33% of women above the 50 suffer from various heart problems. Whereas, only 26% of men over the age of 50 suffer from heart problems. The problem doesn't end here.

There is scientific data to suggest that women suffering from diabetes have a 50% higher risk of fatality from heart problems than the men of same age groups suffering from both these conditions.

What Does This Data Mean?

This data suggests that longevity poses a different set of problems for women.

Although women have a comparatively longer lifespan than men, they are at a greater risk of chronic illnesses and comorbidities like obesity, high blood pressure, diabetes, metabolic syndrome, heart problems, thyroid issues, PCOS, kidney, and liver diseases, etc.

Youth and beauty are two very important things for every woman in the world. However, as we age, along with beauty, health also becomes a very important priority. Women are prone to chronic illnesses, and hence health starts to fail them as they age. Hence, they must work on improving their health as they age.

Chronic illnesses have a very scary characteristic. They remain dormant and keep developing silently inside the body. By the time you are young, there are very few symptoms of chronic illnesses that you may experience. When the body is young and energetic, it is easy to ignore the symptoms and keep working normally. The symptoms of most chronic illnesses can be misinterpreted easily, and hence it is easily possible that they remain undetected till a very advanced stated. But, all this would become a serious problem at an advancing age.

As women reach 50, they are crossing the prime of their health. Till this age, most chronic illnesses don't show significant symptoms.

For instance, insulin resistance is one of the most common health issues. At present more than 80 million adults in the US are suffering from this problem. It is also known as prediabetes, and it leads to glucose tolerance problems. However, you may have insulin resistance for one or two decades and may never feel the need to get tested for it. The mechanism of our body keeps struggling with the problem for a very long but if you don't care, it will lose and finally, the problem of insulin resistance or prediabetes would turn into diabetes.

Chronic health issues don't arise alone. They give rise to other health issues too. For example, if a person has insulin resistance, the risk of obesity increases many times. It would also lead to high blood pressure. Insulin resistance can also cause high cholesterol.

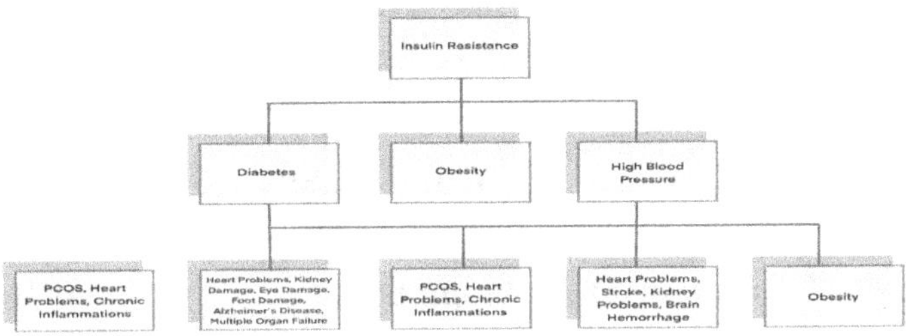

In the figure given above, you can see how one chronic issue can lead to another problem, and then it takes the form of a chain reaction.

Precaution Is Better Than Cure

Some old sayings never get out of fashion, and even this is one among them. The chronic illnesses once make their way into your body; they are very hard to get rid of. It is always best to prevent their development. It is even more important for women over 50 as they are likely to live longer and also more vulnerable to these chronic illnesses due to certain gender-specific hormonal issues.

We all make provisions all our lives to live the final part of our journey with greater comfort and happiness. After infancy, this is the most vulnerable age. Chronic illnesses can make life very difficult at this age once the body falls prey to them.

Data suggests that you might not have any reason to doubt these facts. A report presented by the National Conference of State Legislatures (NCSL) in 2015 states that every year more than 1.7 million people lose their lives due to chronic illnesses. If these numbers don't tell anything, then you'll be surprised to know that women comprise more than 80% of these fatalities. Not only this, but 7 out of 10 deaths in women have one of the chronic illnesses as an underlying cause of death.

As far as women are concerned, they face some unique challenges. The report suggests that more than 38% of women in their advancing age have more than one chronic illness.

There is no denying the fact that age adversely affects all. However, the facts correctly demonstrate that women are especially more vulnerable in their advancing age as they have a comparatively longer lifespan and a greater chance of having chronic illnesses. Therefore, it becomes even more important for them to remain more conscious and cautious about their health.

Chronic Illnesses

Till now, we have discussed a lot about the impact of chronic illnesses. Let us now discuss chronic illnesses and why they are so important.

We must always remain aware of the enemies we can't see. They are even deadlier than the ones that are always fighting with you as you are almost defenseless against an unknown enemy.

Medical science has made tremendous progress. We have found a cure for most illnesses. Even attaching completely severed limbs is easily possible. It is possible to reconstruct a fully damaged face. Even fighting cancer is possible to a great extent. Yet, a simply flu-like virus has been able to bring the whole world to its knees.

Is it not surprising that the first world countries like the US, UK, Italy, Spain, Germany, and France are not able to fight the CoVID-

19 Coronavirus. Even a country like China, which had the full might of the state, had to come to a standstill to contain the virus.

It is not the virus that's the problem. There are vaccines for even deadlier viruses. The 2003 SARS and 2012 MERS infections had much higher fatality rates. But we know their causes, origins, and cure, and hence we are not afraid of them anymore. The COVID-19 is still fairly new and unknown and hence it is more dangerous.

The same is the case with chronic illnesses. They develop in the background. Most of the time, you will have no symptom, and one of the vital functions would start performing poorly. If you don't take any corrective action, which you can't because you don't know which action to take, the problem would blow out of proportion in some time and cause serious damage.

Chronic illnesses can be very dangerous as they put their full weight on your system and make the functioning of the system difficult. A chronic illness like high blood pressure or diabetes will not just have a direct impact, but it will start damaging the systems left, right, and center.

Therefore, you must pay attention to these chronic illnesses and check their progress on time. Letting them go out of hand can be very dangerous as these problems have no cure. For the rest of your life, you can only take medications to manage these illnesses, and that can become very difficult.

The Cause of Chronic Illnesses

Chronic illnesses are a result of system malfunction. These illnesses occur because, most likely, we have been behaving badly with our bodies. They are a result of poor lifestyle.

This should not come as a surprise because most of us know this basic fact that chronic illnesses are a result of a poor lifestyle. Unhealthy food choices, poor eating habits, and a sedentary lifestyle are some of the common reasons our system starts performing poorly.

Even the biggest problems in the body like diabetes begin with simple irregularity in eating habits. Your blood pressure problem can just be a result of a lack of physical activity, excessive salt intake, or even obesity.

Chronic illnesses don't emerge as big problems. They start slow. Like diabetes begins as a glucose tolerance issue. Your body sends you several signals like obesity, high blood pressure, high cholesterol, and PCOS; it is your unwillingness to hear the signals which finally results in diabetes.

Significance For Women?

Women must pay special attention to chronic illnesses while still there is time to do so. Chronic illnesses can destroy the pillars on which they are trying to base their happiness in the future.

For most of a woman's active life, beauty, youth, and charm remain the focus of everything. As they start reaching their 50s, signs of aging start appearing. The problems that meant nothing for them till then or the problems which their bodies could easily ignore till then start emerging as real issues. This is the time when the attention starts to fade, and the problems begin emerging and women are left fending for themselves.

Chronic illnesses can also bring about early signs of aging and a slew of other health problems.

The biggest problem with chronic illnesses is that they don't develop overnight, and hence getting rid of them in a jiffy isn't possible. Fighting chronic illnesses can be a long, tiring, and gruesome battle.

Medicines can help you in managing the symptoms of chronic illnesses, but they don't offer permanent relief. You will have to remain dependent on medication for the rest of your life if you want to take that route.

The best way to ease the symptoms of reverse chronic illnesses is to bring lifestyle changes. Most people fail to realize that it was the poor lifestyle that got them into the problem in the first place. If they bring changes to their poor lifestyle, they can see significant improvement in their chronic illnesses.

Intermittent Fasting and Chronic Illnesses

Intermittent fasting is a simple and easy way to bring a positive change in your lifestyle that can help you in making your life better. Health is the most important wealth you are going to carry in the coming years of your life. No wealth can be enjoyed if you don't enjoy good health. Intermittent fasting is a way to help you attain good health easily.

It is a simple and amazing lifestyle change that can help you in achieving and maintaining great health with considerable ease. It is easy to follow, less restrictive than usual weight loss methods or diets, very effective, and free of cost.

Intermittent fasting is a lifestyle that can fit into anyone's lifestyle, and it can work wonders for women above 50.

Intermittent Is Just Not a Weight Loss Method; It Is a Holistic Health Concept

In the recent past, intermittent fasting has emerged as a popular way to lose weight rapidly. Most women are trying to learn intermittent fasting as they want to get rid of their weight. They are losing on a very big opportunity because if followed properly, intermittent fasting can also help them in getting great health all the while they lose their weight safely. It is an amazing way to reverse chronic illnesses.

Intermittent fasting is particularly a great health concept for women over 50 as they can follow it safely without most of the restrictions applied to younger women due to their hormonal imbalances.

If followed properly, intermittent fasting will not only help them lose weight, look slim, but it would also reverse the signs of aging. By following intermittent fasting, you will not only be able to look much younger but would also feel the same as it helps in energizing your system from inside.

One of the biggest drawbacks of a poor lifestyle is that it overloads the system with a lot of toxins. Poor eating habits, unhealthy food, and a sedentary lifestyle can make the body react poorly even to the right stimuli. Intermittent fasting would help you in overcoming all these problems easily.

Help You in Preparing Better

As we age, we realize that the later part of life is not going to be as easy as we thought it to be. Even simple chores can become difficult with failing health.

As we have already seen, the stats suggest that women are more likely to live longer and that too alone. This is also the time that chronic illnesses would also start raising their head.

Intermittent fasting is simply a way to counter all these issues with some very simple, practical, and actionable solutions.

This book will help you in understanding those solutions and the ways to implement them in your life so that you can enjoy your life in a much better way.

This book will explain how intermittent fasting can work for you and the benefits you can get from it. This book will also explain the ways to maximize your gains to improve your health considerably.

Intermittent fasting is very simple and easy to understand lifestyle change.

I hope that you will be able to get the benefit of this amazing lifestyle!

CHAPTER 2

KEY CHRONIC HEALTH ISSUES WOMEN FACE AFTER 50

Before we dive deep into intermittent fasting, let us have a brief look at some common health issues faced by women once they cross their 50s and their impact.

Obesity

Obesity is the most common and even the most glaring concern women of all age groups in America have. Rightly, it should be a great concern as 7 out of 10 American adults are either overweight or obese. Even in this, the women are ahead of men. CDC report states that out of all the cases, 37.9% of all the men were obese. This was found to be 41.1% in women.

We all know that obesity has taken the form of an epidemic. More than 2 adults out of 3 suffering from the problem can't be classified in any other way. However, the approach of people towards obesity is wrong.

Even today, most people, especially women, consider obesity to be a mere cosmetic problem.

In the US, every year, there are around 900,000 preventable deaths. These are the deaths that could have been prevented if the patients had been a bit more vigilant about their health and vital parameters. Out of these around 500,000 deaths have obesity as one of the underlying causes.

These are scary stats as they suggest that obesity can be a reason for a lot of health problems. This is a conclusion that most people have drawn, and that's why there is such a great rush to get rid of obesity. So many diets and weight loss treatments are a result of this thinking.

However, this is an incorrect presumption. Obesity is not the cause of all the health issues you are facing but a sign that the vital functions in your body have started to get compromised.

Being fat in itself can be a cosmetic issue. You may not fit into some clothes or may feel awkward in social circles, but it is not a health issue in itself. It is the reason you get obese that must be the cause of your concern. You will have to understand that you simply can't get fat because you are consuming a few extra calories. Obesity is a result of a malfunction of the way your body processes energy.

One can get obese due to hormonal imbalances, insulin resistance, poor metabolism, thyroid malfunction, and many such issues, and the underlying problems that arise due to the circumstances would create a health emergency.

Data also states that the rate of obesity is much higher as you reach your 50s than what it was compared to your 30s. This happens because your overall metabolism and the energy processing mechanism slows down. The body also develops conditions like insulin resistance, PCOS, thyroid, and other hormonal issues and hence, the weight starts to rise rapidly.

Obesity is a very important health issue that women must acknowledge in the right way. The bulging fat at the abdomen, thighs, and hips is just not something that may be causing wardrobe inconveniences, but it is also leading to many health issues.

Obesity can lead to chronic inflammations, high cholesterol, poor heart function, high blood pressure, poor fertility, hormone imbalances, and many other such issues.

It is also one of the most common health issues faced by women as they reach their 50s. As the age advances, several crucial functions like insulin sensitivity, leptin sensitivity, and metabolism get compromised, which may lead to a rapid increase in weight. Overcoming obesity must at the top of your agenda list if you want to lead a healthy life in your 50s and reduce the risk of chronic illnesses.

We all know that obesity is primarily caused by lifestyle disorders. A poor lifestyle and your diet can play a very important role in managing your weight properly. However, many women fail to bring any change in their weight even after employing several weight loss measures. Even if they do achieve some weight loss, the weight relapse is almost certain and even more than before.

Intermittent fasting can provide you a reliable solution to these problems. It is a simple and effective way to modify your way of living that can help in rapid weight loss easily.

Diabetes

Diabetes is another very serious health risk faced by women in their 50s. As per the CDC reports, more than 30 million adults in the US suffer from diabetes. It is a debilitating illness as it restricts your life to a great extent. It takes away your liberties. From the things you can eat to when and how you can eat, have to be monitored carefully. Diabetes is a dangerous condition as it can lead to heart problems, multiple organ failures, skin conditions, eye damage, foot damage, high blood pressure, and obesity.

Not only this, but the risk of diabetes is also much higher in women. Reports also suggest that women with diabetes are at a 50% higher risk of heart attacks than men in the same age group suffering from diabetes.

Even alarming is the fact that the 30 million people who are suffering from diabetes only form one part of the story. Another 80 million people are battling with prediabetes in the US. This condition is the precursor to diabetes. If steps are not taken on time, the chances of prediabetes turning into diabetes are very high.

Women in their 50s are highly affected by this condition, and they are also most likely to fall prey to diabetes. For them, it becomes even more important to find ways to reverse prediabetes or else several other illnesses will get hold on their body.

Intermittent fasting can prove to be a great book for women over 50 as it can help them in reversing insulin resistance that can help them in preventing the onset of diabetes. Intermittent fasting is one of the best ways to improve insulin sensitivity that can help in the reversal of prediabetes and the prevention of diabetes.

High Blood Pressure

High blood pressure or hypertension is a common health condition affecting millions of women. As per the American Heart Association's (AHA) statistics published in 2018, more than 103 million Americans suffer from high blood pressure. Out of these, more than half are women.

Another study conducted by NCHS brings out a trend that a fewer number of women suffer from high blood pressure as compared to men in their 20s and 30s. Between the age group of 20-34, around 9.1% of men suffered from high blood pressure, whereas the percentage of women suffering from the same was 6.7. Even in the 35-44 age group, around 37.7 men suffered from high blood pressure whereas the percentage of women suffering from the same is 34.

However, this trend changes as age advances. In the 50s, around 52% of men and women suffer from high blood pressure, and in the 60s, more than 70% of women suffer from high blood pressure while the percentage of men suffering from the same is 63.

Studies show that one in three deaths in women is caused by cardiovascular diseases and high blood pressure is at the base of these.

High blood pressure is also a lifestyle disorder that can be caused by several issues like obesity, insulin resistance, poor diet, high salt intake, and unhealthy lifestyle. Out of these, obesity and insulin resistance are two main reasons that can lead to high blood pressure.

Intermittent fasting can help you in fighting the chief reasons that can lead to high blood pressure. It is a condition that can not only lead to heart problems, but it can also cause severe damage to your kidneys as well as may also lead to brain hemorrhage.

Cardiovascular Diseases

Women are soft-hearted. This is taken as a compliment all over the world. However, women are also known for their weakness in heart diseases. Heart problems are among the highest killers in women.

CDC reports say that every year more than 293,000 women lose their lives due to heart attacks itself. This is a very big number.

Heart problems are not very pleasant in any case, but even before they claim the lives of the victims, they can practically bring life to a standstill. From various diet restrictions, excessive medication, movement restrictions to other limitations, heart problems can make the life of a patient very difficult.

The biggest blame for heart problems is put on cholesterol. However, that's not the whole truth.

Studies have proven that dietary cholesterol has little role to play in the health of the heart. The cholesterol that clogs the arteries is produced in the liver itself. Obesity, high blood sugar levels, and insulin resistance are among the biggest causes of high cholesterol in your body.

Not only this, but high blood sugar levels and high blood pressure cause the highest amount of ischemic injuries in many ways that finally lead to heart attacks.

As we have already discussed, all these issues are lifestyle disorders, and hence they can be resolved effectively with the help of intermittent fasting.

The practice of intermittent fasting can practically help you in bringing down the triglyceride levels in your body. It is the most dangerous kind of cholesterol for your heart. Intermittent fasting also helps in lowering bad cholesterols like LDL and VLDL.

Therefore, practicing intermittent fasting can give your heart a new lease of life, and you will be able to feel a great improvement in your overall health.

Polycystic Ovarian Syndrome (PCOS)

Of all the problems faced by women, this one is specific to them. Polycystic Ovarian Syndrome or PCOS, as it is popularly known only affects women. However, that doesn't mean it is lenient in its severity.

In the US, more than 5 million women are currently suffering from this condition. At the global level, this number is as high as 114 million. It is a condition that affects the ovaries and the complete reproductive system of women. However, its impact is just not limited to that.

PCOS causes several hormonal imbalances in the body of a woman. Insulin resistance, obesity, metabolic dysfunction, thyroid, and chronic inflammations can be a few among them.

Girls can get affected by this condition as soon as they hit puberty, and it can affect women of all age groups. Although women who have attained menopause can't get affected by PCOS, this doesn't mean that women who have PCOS will stop getting affected by it once they reach menopause. On the contrary, PCOS along with other comorbidities like high blood pressure, diabetes, heart problems, and chronic inflammations, can make the lives of women even more difficult in the advancing age.

Many women also have the misconception that if the ovaries are surgically removed, they can get rid of PCOS because it is an ovarian disease. They are also wrong because although the name of this disease is a polycystic ovarian syndrome, in reality, it begins in the brain. Even the removal of ovaries will not provide any relief and women who have been suffering from PCOS will keep facing the symptoms.

PCOS is primarily a hormonal dysfunction in women that takes place in the pituitary gland in the brain. It can cause an imbalance in the release of several other hormones too.

There is no direct way to control the release of hormones in the brain. However, with the help of a balanced lifestyle provided by intermittent fasting, you can reduce the severity of PCOS.

Intermittent fasting can help in lowering associated conditions like insulin resistance, obesity, high blood pressure, and chronic inflammations. As these issues subside, women feel more at ease, and they can enjoy their lives better.

Osteoarthritis

This is another big problem faced by women in various forms. The weakness of bones, joint problems, and other such issues can make the life of women very difficult in their advancing age.

Our body has a system to make new bone cells in place of worn down cells. However, this process takes a hit after you reach your 50s. By this time, the body becomes incapable of replacing the worn down cells at the pace at which they are dying. This means that the bones become weaker, and hence bone injuries become commonplace.

Chronic inflammations also find their ways to affect your bones and joints, and arthritis emerges as a common issue.

Poor lifestyle and deficient diet along with chronic inflammations, are responsible for these conditions. With the help of an intermittent lifestyle, you can expect a great improvement in this area.

CHAPTER 3

THE WAY POOR LIFESTYLE IS RESPONSIBLE FOR MOST CHRONIC ILLNESSES

All through our youth, we all know that in some way or the other, a poor lifestyle will lead to ill health. We repeatedly get advised to mend our ways by the doctors, health professionals, and health experts besides our elders. Yet, we fail to pay heed to those advises as we don't observe any immediate side effect of our unhealthy practices the next day or in the short-term.

Chronic illnesses are nothing else but a malfunction in our vital systems. Our blood circulation, blood sugar management, blood refining process, blood pumping system, and energy storage mechanism are the vital functions that need to run smoothly for a healthy body.

These processes are crucial for our whole system, and that's why they are very resilient. You can't shake these systems through a day of callousness. It takes years and years of undoing to make these functions perform poorly.

In this chapter, we will try to understand how a poor lifestyle can affect the functioning of vital processes.

The Blood Sugar Management Process

Blood sugar management is among the most crucial functions in the body. It is the process through which your cells get energy, and they can perform their function.

If the blood sugar management process in your body stops performing properly, your cells would start starving. No matter the kind of food you eat, your cells would stop getting energy. This would also create blood sugar management issues because if the cells don't absorb energy, the glucose in the blood would become a problem in itself.

Several things can cause damage to the blood sugar management system:

Poor Sugar-laden Diet: Modern American diet is laden with sugar and refined products. Sweetened beverages like sodas, flavored drinks, and alcoholic beverages have become the mainstay of our lifestyles. However, these things do nothing else than causing frequent insulin spikes in our blood. They keep our blood sugar levels high, and our blood sugar management system keeps struggling with the issue. While you are young, the system is robust and it struggles with its full might. However, as you age, the system slows down and you start facing problems like insulin resistance, low energy, lethargy, diabetes, and obesity.

Poor Eating Habits: The way we eat these days, it is nothing short of grazing tendency. We don't eat because we feel hungry. On the contrary, we eat because we find an opportunity to eat, we see a food stall with something tempting on it.

- We eat because we feel that our stomach is empty.
- We eat because we are not feeling happy.
- We also eat when we are feeling very happy to celebrate.
- We tend to eat when we are discussing business.
- We like to eat when we are chatting with our friends.
- We eat when we feel that we are getting bored.
- We like to eat when we are getting entertained sitting in front of a TV screen or a movie theatre, or even a game.

Eating has become our most favorite pastime. However, this excessive and frequent eating not only adds extra calories and overloads our digestive system, but it also affects our blood sugar management system.

Every time you consume food, the digestive system breaks it down and converts it into energy. This energy is passed on to the system in the form of glucose.

As this glucose mixes into your blood, your blood sugar levels increase. This glucose is very important. The cells in your body can use this glucose directly in this form itself. It doesn't require any further processing, and hence they can get instant energy. However, the cells can't absorb this glucose without help. They need insulin signals.

Insulin is a hormone produced by the beta cells in your pancreas. This is a very important hormone that is the backbone of the whole energy metabolization process.

As soon as you consume calories in any form, the pancreas senses the rise in blood sugar levels and starts releasing insulin to facilitate glucose absorption by the cells.

The insulin receptors in the cells identify the insulin signals and open up to absorb glucose. This process facilitates glucose absorption by the cells in the body, and it also helps in lowering the blood sugar levels.

Ideally, this process should take place two-three times a day. However, as per our current lifestyle and eating patterns, we tend to eat several times a day, causing insulin spikes multiple times. This causes overexposure of insulin to the cells and their response to the insulin signal gets slow. This means the whole glucose absorption system becomes slow and inefficient. Most of the time, the cells are not even able to absorb the amount of glucose they need. This leads to lethargy, fatigue, weakness, and lack of energy.

However, the problem doesn't come to an end here itself. Because the cells are not absorbing glucose readily, the blood sugar levels tend to remain abnormally high for unreasonable periods. This can be lethal as high blood sugar levels can lead to high blood pressure, thickening of blood vessels, pressure on the vital organs like the heart, kidneys, and the liver.

The insulin is also the key fat storage hormone in the body, and hence whatever blood sugar is left after the absorption of the cells, it is stored in the body as glycogen and fat. However, insulin resistance shown by the cells can make the process very lengthy. The process of converting glucose to fat is very slow and the insulin should only have only a very small amount of glucose left to do that. But when you start consuming food at very short intervals and the response of the cells slows down considerably, insulin comes face to face with dual problems.

Insulin struggles with the blood sugar management issue, and it starts converting the glucose in the blood directly into triglycerides. This, in turn, increases the triglyceride levels in your blood alarmingly and it can be dangerous for your heart health.

Therefore, you can see that a small thing like frequent consumption of meals can also have a devastating effect on your system. Doing this once in a while may not have any effect on our health, and our body is well equipped to deal with such situations. However, when you make it a habit and keep practicing it for most of your life, your blood sugar management system breaks down.

Poor eating habits will lead to insulin resistance, obesity, poor blood sugar management, high cholesterol, high triglyceride levels, diabetes, and high chronic inflammation.

A Sedentary Lifestyle: Our lifestyle also plays a very crucial role in our health. If you are living an active lifestyle, your energy expenditure would be high, and this would mean that your body will be able to process energy better. Even if you eat more, it would easily get used up and the risk of obesity would be less.

However, if you are leading a very sedentary lifestyle, your energy expenditure would be very less. If you are consuming too many extra calories than your **Basal Metabolic Rate (BMR),** then your body will not be able to use those calories, and they will get stored as fat. This will also lead to obesity. But, obesity will not be the only problem that your body faces if it is already suffering from insulin resistance too. In that case, it would also lead to problems like high toxic waste in the body caused by prolonged exposure to glucose, more fat and cholesterol, chronic inflammation, and other such issues.

Therefore, you can see that a poor lifestyle can have an overbearing effect on your overall health. It doesn't cause a single problem like obesity but has a compounding effect on your health and can make you very ill over a while.

You can see that a poor lifestyle doesn't affect one system exclusively. It has a cascading effect on other systems as well.

Poor eating habits not only lead to insulin resistance, but they also cause obesity. It is also responsible for high triglyceride formation, which leads to heart issues. If left untreated for long, insulin resistance will turn into diabetes too.

Most chronic illnesses originate in the same way. One chronic illness leads to another, and they combine to form metabolic syndrome or syndrome X.

As we have already discussed, medicines in most chronic illnesses can only help you manage the symptoms, but they don't offer a permanent solution.

For example, doctors may give you medicines like Metformin or Victoza to help in diabetes. You may also need to take insulin shots if your blood sugar levels are very high. However, even these medicines can only help in managing your blood sugar levels and will not work on reversing diabetes because it is a process that is malfunctioning from inside.

Another example would be PCOS. It is a common problem in women and there are millions of women suffering from this condition. Yet, until now, there is no medication to cure PCOS. Whatever treatment you might get from your doctor would be symptomatic. If you are not getting your periods, you may be temporarily put on birth control pills. They help in providing the hormones that can help in releasing your eggs. If you are gaining fat rapidly, the doctor may advise you metformin to help you lose weight by managing your insulin resistance. If you have acne or hirsutism, then you would be given separate medication for these symptoms but there is no standard blanket treatment for PCOS.

Even in case of heart problems caused by high cholesterol, the doctors usually prescribe statins to help in lowering the production of lipids in your blood. However, you shouldn't forget the fact that statin doesn't differentiate between good and bad cholesterol. It brings down both. It is a highly popular line of treatment all over the globe, but it is not the perfect treatment. There are several side effects of the medication and it doesn't help the heart much in any particular way. This is the reason doctors prescribe so many lifestyle changes to the heart patients so that the problem can be contained through medication and recovery can be made from lifestyle changes.

Intermittent Fasting Can Be a Key in Reversing Chronic Illnesses

Intermittent fasting is a simple lifestyle change that can help in reversing several chronic illnesses. It is an age-old practice that humankind had been practicing for hundreds of thousands of years. Our bodies have evolved on this system, and hence they work the best with it.

Through the simple method of fasting and eating at certain intervals can help your systems in recovering from years of abuse that you have been subjecting them to. It is a comprehensive way to lose way through the correct method, and that would also help in easing the burden from your body.

Intermittent fasting creates a system where your body can respond better to various changes. It also helps your body in beginning the process of autophagy that can also begin the self-healing process.

Two very important concepts that you will hear in this context are:

1. Ketosis

2. Autophagy

Ketosis: Ketosis is the process of burning fat for energy. Most people trying to lose weight fail to get any success or end up gaining more than they had ever lost. This happens because they hadn't lost any weight in reality. Most of the time, the lost weight is just the water weight that their body loses to adjust to the current energy crisis. To lose real weight, your body would have to begin the process of ketosis. Intermittent fasting can help you in beginning this process fast. Aided with a correct nutrition plan, you can expect ketosis to begin rapidly, and not only will your weight go down but you will also experience fat-burning from your abdomen, thighs, and hips.

Autophagy: It is another term that you might have come across recently if you have been following the health news closely. It is a process of self-cleaning that your body is capable of carrying out under the right conditions. A study on this subject has helped a Japanese researcher win the 2016 Nobel Prize in medicine. This process can unlock the secret of longevity, health, and cure from some of the most untreatable conditions. The research on this subject has brought to light that under correct fasting conditions, the body can start purging all the inefficient processes, pathogens, and useless material inside the body to make it more energy-efficient. This process can help in healing from several illnesses, and it also has strong anti-aging effects.

Both these processes, combined with intermittent fasting, can help you in fighting most of the chronic illnesses in your body to a great extent.

Intermittent fasting is a positive lifestyle change that can help you in reversing the negative impact of chronic illnesses, and you can expect to live your future life in better health.

There are some of the most adamant health issues that we keep struggling with for most of our lives, but see no end to them. Intermittent fasting can also help you in fighting even those issues.

One such problem is obesity. Increasing weight and waistline is among the chief concerns of women of all age groups. However, it becomes a major health concern of women in their 50s as it also starts affecting their overall health.

The first advice health care professionals give to overweight women is to control their weight to stay healthy. However, that's easy said than done.

Weight is adamant, and especially the belly fat simply refuses to go. Women, throughout their lives, try numerous methods but to no avail. Getting rid of weight is a big problem but once you have lost some weight, preventing weight relapse is an even bigger problem.

Statistics show that more than 85% of women who had lost weight eventually regained more than they had lost.

Intermittent fasting can help you in getting freedom from this vicious cycle of gaining and losing weight. You can successfully lose weight and easily maintain it with the help of an intermittent fasting lifestyle.

CHAPTER 4

THE PROBLEM OF WEIGHT RELAPSE AND THE SOLUTION

As we discussed in the previous chapter, the problem of weight relapse is even more serious for women than the initial weight loss.

To understand this issue, you will also have to understand the issue of losing water weight in the right context.

What Is Water Weight?

We all are made up of water. A major portion of our weight comes from water. It runs in our veins in the form of blood. There is a lot of moisture in our tissues. Water is in our body in various forms.

However, our body also retains water in its actual form for various purposes. One of the important functions is to regulate body temperature. You might have observed that people in good health feel less hot or cold as compared to other people who aren't in such good health. It happens because all healthy people have a lot of water in their body, regulating the temperature.

A part of the energy that we get through food is used for this purpose. The more well-fed or well-nourished and healthy you are, the more comfortable you are likely to feel. The reason is simple; your body will have ample energy to spare to make you feel comfortable.

The water that is used for this temperature regulation has its weight. That weight is called water weight.

What Leads to the Loss of Water Weight?

When you begin the process of losing weight, the first thing that you target is the calorie intake. We are repeatedly told that if we eat more calories, we will get fat. Therefore, as per conventional wisdom, we begin by lowering our calorie intake.

The first impact of lower calorie intake is that it creates an energy deficit.

Before we move any further, you must understand the concept of **Basal Metabolic Rate or BMR**.

BMR: Our body has two kinds of energy needs:

1. The Constant Energy Need
2. The Variable Energy Need

The **Constant Energy Need** is the fixed energy requirement of your body to run the crucial functions like blood circulation, the pumping of the heart, the functioning of the kidneys, the liver function, etc.

The body needs to run these processes all the time, even when the person is sleeping or in a medical coma. The energy demand created by such processes is called the BMR. It can be calculated by a specific mathematical formula that keeps into your account your weight, height, gender, and other such things.

This is the minimum energy required by the body to survive even if you are not doing any physical activity. Even if you don't move a muscle, your body would need these many calories.

The **Variable Energy Need** can vary depending upon the kind of physical activity undertaken by you. Energy needs to maintain an active lifestyle would be higher. The same would be lower for a person leading a sedentary lifestyle. In the same way, there are several processes that the body runs when it is in an energy surplus. Those processes have the end goal of providing you comfort. Regulating the body heat against outside temperature is one such comfort energy expenditure.

Whenever you go on a calorie-restrictive diet, your body would need to choose to cut energy from one of the segments. You can rely on the prudence of the body; it will always try to bring down the variable energy needs first.

In this pursuit, when you lower your calorie intake, the body starts looking for areas to cut energy. The first thing to go is temperature regulation. As a result, your body starts dumping excess water rapidly.

If you have ever been on a calorie-restrictive diet, you would appreciate the fact that the weight loss in the initial period is rapid, and it starts plateauing after a few weeks. The reason is simple. Initially, your body is hoarding a lot of water and it starts dumping it rapidly and that's why you see a rapid weight loss. But, as once you have lost your water weight, calorie-restriction cannot help you with weight loss.

Why Calorie-Restriction Is Ineffective in Actual Weight Loss

You would have to appreciate the prudence of the body for that. Most people believe that if they lower the calorie intake below a certain level, the body would start targeting its fat stores for energy. However, even you wouldn't do that in normal circumstances, if you know that there is going to be a shortage of something. Rationing is in our very nature.

When you lower your calorie intake, the body first tries to lower its variable energy needs. However, there is a limit to that. If you have an active lifestyle, even when your calorie intake is low, your variable energy needs would remain high. You may feel tired more often but you will still keep getting the required energy.

In such a case, the body would start to look for areas to lower its constant energy needs. When many animals go in hibernation, their heartbeats become slow. Their whole metabolic process slows down so that they can survive on the same amount of energy for much longer. The body starts doing the same with the BMR.

In the case of a strict Calorie-Deficient diet, you may feel tired more often. There can be a feeling of lethargy and unwillingness to do anything. All these are subtle hints being dropped by the body to lower the energy expenditure.

If you'd appreciate it, you'd notice that till now, there is no mention of the body making any effort to use the energy stored in the form of fat.

You must remember that the body would only come for stored energy only when the outside energy supply comes to a halt and not when it becomes low or slow.

This is the biggest reason people don't experience fat-burning by simply following a calorie-restrictive diet.

The calorie-restrictive diets can be very punishing as they limit the food intake to a great extent. The body is starving for food. This is the reason most women have very strong food cravings when they are on diets.

The diets can only be for a specific period. Once you get off a diet, you would have very strong food temptations. This leads to binge eating, and the weight comes back even faster than you had lost it.

The Reason for Weight Relapse

Most women think that if they don't eat too much, they won't face weight relapse. However, they get disappointed and even with a very restricted calorie intake, they start experiencing weight gain.

It is incorrect to think that you will only lose weight when you eat a lot. It is not the food but the amount of energy going inside you that will lead to weight gain.

As soon as you resume eating the required number of calories, there is no need for the body to not begin the process of heat regulation. It begins retaining the water once again, and hence you see a rapid rise in your weight.

You must understand that weight lost or gained in a short period is water weight. It is not the weight lost by the body due to the burning of actual body fat.

Burning of body fat is a very complex process, and it can only happen in a specific set of conditions that we will discuss in the next chapter and the point where intermittent fasting comes into the picture.

CHAPTER 5

BURNING FAT WITH INTERMITTENT FASTING

Weight loss has emerged as a billion-dollar industry. It had a market valuation of over 70 billion last year. This is for an industry that didn't even exist a few decades back. The world didn't recognize obesity as a mainstream problem a century ago. Back then, malnutrition was a real problem. However, the circumstances have changed.

Today, obesity is a problem affecting more than 1.9 billion people all over the globe. However, have you ever wondered the reason most people fail to lose weight?

Weight loss is such a big problem because people don't address the correct issue.

Calories Are Not the Cause of Weight Gain

A very big misconception people have in their minds is that a few extra calories are the sole reason for their weight gain. They are wrong. Period.

Burning stored body fat is a much more complex process than you think. Until you don't understand the process, you will keep failing at losing weight and burning body fat.

But, before that, you will have to understand that fat is important for the body and it fights tooth and nail to conserve this fat.

The Importance of Fat for the Body

Have you ever wondered the reason it is so difficult to burn body fat? It is so difficult because the body values this fat highly, and it tries everything in its might to protect it.

You know that we have passed through millions of years of an evolutionary process. This process has given the basic learning that the times are always not the same. Periods of feasts and famines keep alternating. This means the species that is not prepared for long fasting periods or periods of famine will not last very long.

That's why every species has its mechanism to survive long-fasting periods. The body fat is our very own mechanism to get through periods of famine.

Our body keeps collecting energy from almost every meal that we have and stores it as fat. It protects this fat aggressively because it knows that in a condition of complete energy cut-off, only this fat can help the body survive for the longest.

This is one of the reasons your body wouldn't start burning fat at the first instant of lower energy intake.

However, this is not the only reason your body doesn't begin burning fat immediately. There are two more reasons.

Other Two Important Factors for Burning Fat

To burn fat, only the energy deficit is not a sufficient ground. Two more things will be required to burn fat. The first is readiness, and the second is the mode.

Let us understand both in detail:

Lack of Readiness- Insulin Resistance: As we had previously discussed, besides being the facilitator of glucose absorption, insulin is also the key fat-storage hormone. Whatever glucose is left in the bloodstream after the absorption of the cells, insulin stores it in the muscles, liver, and fat tissues.

How Fat Storage Works

The glucose in the bloodstream keeps the blood sugar levels high, and that can be dangerous for the functioning of the vital organs. It can also affect crucial functions like blood pressure and elasticity of the muscles. The high blood sugar content can harden the vessels and they'll become prone to damage. That's the reason it is the job of insulin to lower the blood sugar levels rapidly.

This can be done fastest through absorption by the cells.

However, whatever glucose is left in the bloodstream, insulin starts storing it as glycogen in the muscles. But, the muscles can't store a lot of it. As soon as the muscle glycogen stores are full, insulin starts storing glucose as glycogen in the liver.

The liver can store a substantial amount of energy. Your body can run only on the glycogen stored in the liver for almost 36 hours.

However, the glycogen stores of the liver keep filling up regularly, and hence insulin will not get to store a lot there.

The last place to store all the excess glucose is in the adipose tissues. A lot of fat can be stored as subcutaneous fat under your belly, thighs, and hips.

The Detrimental Impact of Insulin Resistance

As you know that insulin is a very important hormone, and it performs several crucial functions. Two key functions are facilitating glucose absorption by the cells and fat storage.

When your cells become insulin resistant, both these functions get affected.

First of all, the cells respond slowly to the insulin signals, and hence your blood sugar levels remain high for longer than required. Due to this, the pancreas starts pumping more insulin as it wants the blood sugar levels to go down. However, more insulin is not solving the problem. More insulin means more exposure to the cells which are already battling overexposure. This escalates the problem further.

This means that the cells wouldn't be in a condition to readily accept glucose, and the blood sugar levels would remain high. To solve this problem, insulin has no other option than to rapidly convert glucose into fat.

Now, as we have already discussed, insulin is the key fat-storage hormone. As long as there is a high insulin presence in your bloodstream, your body would remain in a fat-storage mode.

Once released by the pancreas, it takes anywhere between 8-12 hours for the insulin levels to go down. Because your body is battling insulin resistance, the insulin levels would be abnormally high because the pancreas keeps pumping more and more insulin.

This also means that your body would remain in a fat storage mode as the insulin levels are unlikely to go down in your body. From your last meal to the next meal, it takes anywhere between 8-12 hours for your insulin levels to go down. If you consume anything between this period, your insulin levels would again shoot up, and your body would stop burning any kind of fat.

Most of us never get that kind of a gap between our meals due to our erratic eating habits. This is one of the chief reasons your body is unlikely to get into a fat-burning mode in normal conditions.

Our erratic habit of eating at short intervals is one of the main culprits of insulin resistance and the resulting obesity. You must keep in mind that as long as your body is insulin resistant, it will struggle with burning fat.

Ketosis- The Fat Burning Mode: Another important reason for failure to burn fat is the wrong fuel mode.

Our body can run on two fuel types:

1. The glucose fuel
2. The fat fuel

You get glucose from the carbs and protein that you consume in your meals. The fat comes from the fat in the meat, fatty fruits, egg yolk, fatty fish, oils, etc.

Your body can easily run on both types of fuel. However, it can't run on both at the same time.

When we are trying to lose weight with the calorie-restriction method or low-calorie diets, we are effectively trying to do just that. We lower the calorie and expect the body to burn fat and glucose at the same time.

This is not going to happen, and it never does. This is the reason most people never burn any real fat despite their best efforts.

As we have discussed, the process of burning fat is called ketosis. In this process, your body switches from glucose fuel to the fat fuel. Once the body has made the switch, and it is only getting fat fuel to burn, it will easily start burning the body fat as fuel.

However, for this to take place, you will have to stop the intake of glucose fuel. This means that you will have to stop the intake of carbs and would also have to manage your protein intake strictly as excess protein would also get converted into glucose, ultimately through the process of glucogenesis.

Burning Fat in Reality

If you want to burn fat, you will have to ensure that there is no excess insulin floating in your bloodstream. You will have to keep this in mind that no matter what, as long as there is insulin in your bloodstream, your body wouldn't start burning fat as it would remain in a fat storage mode.

This is where intermittent fasting is of special use.

Intermittent fasting is the process of creating prolonged gaps between your meals. With the help of intermittent fasting, you will be able to create longer gaps so that the insulin levels can go down very long. In such circumstances, your body would be able to burn fat for energy.

Intermittent fasting is also the best way to lower insulin resistance, and hence you can also expect your cells to become more sensitive to insulin signals. This means that there will be less insulin in your bloodstream if your cells are responding well to the insulin signals.

Intermittent fasting also creates long gaps of glucose absence. Glucose is a short-lived form of energy. This means that your cells can use glucose rapidly. It provides instant energy, but it doesn't last very long. Hence, if you are more insulin sensitive your cells would absorb glucose rapidly and use it up fast.

If you consume food again after a short interval, your body would start facing energy shortage. In the complete absence of glucose, your body can also begin the process of ketosis in which it starts breaking fats to convert them into ketones that can be used as energy.

A fat-rich diet like a ketogenic diet, also called the keto diet, will expedite the process.

The fat that you consume in your diet doesn't get processed in the same way as glucose. It is broken down in the intestines with the help of bile juices released by the gall-bladder.

The bile juices help in breaking the fat into smaller parts, and these are then metabolized in the liver.

However, unlike glucose, you don't need insulin to facilitate the absorption of the ketones by the cells. To facilitate the absorption of ketones, the alpha cells in the pancreas releases glucagon. Hence, there is no insulin response at all in your body. This means that your body will be capable of burning the body fat right away too, if there is any significant need for energy like during heavy exercise.

Therefore, it is with the help of intermittent fasting and a keto diet that you can easily achieve fat-burning much faster and more effectively than any other process.

It is one of the most reliable ways to lose weight rapidly.

You would lose a significant amount of your actual body fat without having to follow a punishing diet or calorie-restriction program. Intermittent fasting is the most scientific way to lose significant weight without compromising your health.

CHAPTER 6

HORMONAL HEALTH OF WOMEN- THE MOST IGNORED FACTOR IN WEIGHT LOSS

One of the most dangerous things that women do while they are trying to lose weight is that they ignore the importance of their hormonal health.

One of the most significant differences between men and women is the way their bodies treat food.

The body of a man doesn't attach too much significance to food. For men, food is just a way to survive. This is in stark contrast to the way the body of a woman treats food.

For women, food means much more than simple survival; it is connected to their hormonal balance.

Since the time a girl hits puberty to the time she reaches menopause, her body is physically always in a readiness mode to bear a child. Bearing a child is a big responsibility. A child in the womb is a big drain on the energy sources in a woman's body. Once a woman conceives a child, her body tries its best to provide nutrition to the child. This was always not possible through conventional mediums in the past.

In the past, women sometimes got food and most of the time didn't. This can make the survival of the child in the womb difficult. To solve this problem, nature has devised the plan of energy store inside the body to help the child survive.

This is the reason women have a comparatively higher body fat ratio than men, and they are also more likely to gain fat rapidly. It is not a weakness they have, but a brilliant plan devised by nature for the survival of the coming generations.

Food and Female Hormones Are Connected

The hormones in the body are chemical messengers that help in passing on vital information to the brain. Hormones regulate several crucial functions. If you look closely, the life of a woman is completely dominated by these hormones.

Thyroid and pituitary are two very important glands that secrete most of the hormones. They also regulate the behavior of a woman. These glands are also present in men but don't have that profound impact on them simply because they are not going to bear a child.

Women feel a very strong connection with food and that's why emotional eating, impulsive eating, celebration eating, and all other forms of eating have such strong meanings for women. For women, food is a part of emotional security as it also helps in the regulation and balancing of certain hormones.

Impact of Calorie-Restrictive Diets of Hormonal Balance

Calorie-restrictive diets can harm the hormonal balance in women. It can fill them with a sense of insecurity, void, and unhappiness. Scientific experiments on mice have shown that prolonged calorie-restriction can also lead to the shrinking of female reproductive organs, and they may also lose their ability to reproduce effectively.

Strict diets can also cause irregular periods, and they may also face problems in conception. Women on calorie-restrictive diets can also experience strong and sudden mood swings and they may also become more temperamental. Anger, frustration, irritation, hopelessness, temptation, and cravings are some of the strong feelings experienced by women when they are on calorie-restrictive diets.

Hormonal Balance is Important

It is very important to understand that hormonal balance is very important. Without the hormonal balance, the overall health of a woman will always remain compromised. This is the problem most women keep facing all their lives.

In the pursuit of weight loss and a slender body, women compromise on their hormonal health and end up paying in the form of problems like PCOS, thyroid, metabolic disorders, and other reproductive issues.

Intermittent Fasting- A Reliable Way to Lose Weight Without Compromising Hormonal Health

Intermittent fasting is a safe way to lose weight as it doesn't force you to compromise with your hormonal health. Intermittent fasting doesn't make you starve for food or limit your calorie intake specifically.

It is a process that allows you to eat reasonably. There are no calorie-restrictions. You can eat whatever you feel like as long as you maintain adequate control over quantity.

This eliminates cravings, temptations, and obsessiveness regarding certain food items, and hence your hormones remain in control.

Intermittent fasting is not about what to eat but when to eat. The most important thing in intermittent fasting is to observe abstinence from food for a certain number of hours every day. This period can be easily timed to be your sleep time, and hence severe hunger pangs, and cravings can easily be avoided.

CHAPTER 7

INTERMITTENT FASTING- THE IDEAL WAY OF LIFE FOR WOMEN OVER 50

50s can be very confusing. This is not the age one qualifies to be a senior neither it is an age where you can relax as the young ones do.

It is the time when you are rapidly inching close to chronic illnesses. Your immunity will get weaker. Your bone health would start deteriorating. There will be signs of aging all around.

Diets, calorie-restriction methods, and other such tools become useless as you want something more sustainable.

Intermittent fasting is one of the most reliable ways to stay healthy and fit as it helps you in staying healthy from the inside. It helps in improving your overall health biomarkers like insulin sensitivity, blood pressure, blood sugar levels, cholesterol levels, chronic inflammations, and satiety and hunger levels too.

The Practice of Intermittent Fasting

The practice of intermittent fasting is very simple.

It divides your day into two parts

1. The Fasting period
2. The Feasting period

The Fasting Period: The fasting period, as the name suggests, would be the time when you will observe complete abstinence from food. During this period, you shouldn't consume anything that has calories. This would also include caloric beverages and snacks. The fasting window can be anywhere between 12-20 hours for women.

Generally, this window is kept short for young girls, as fasting for longer periods can harm their hormonal cycles. However, for women over 50, this doesn't pose a very big problem. On the contrary, slightly longer fasts in this age group can help you in improving your health biomarkers better.

The fasting window is normally kept in the night because passing the fasting time during sleep is easier.

Beginning the fast as early in the evening as possible is the best as it would give you a few extra hours to remain in the fasted state without feeling acute hunger.

The Feasting Period: This is the period when you can have your regular 2-3 meals. The feasting window in intermittent fasting can be as liberal as you wish. This means that intermittent fasting doesn't put specific restrictions on quantity and type of food.

The focus of intermittent fasting is on improving issues like insulin resistance, hormonal imbalances, and chronic inflammations as other things begin improving on their own. Hence, even with slightly larger meal portions, you can keep losing weight consistently.

Eating a keto diet can help you in expediting the ketosis process, and hence your results would begin appearing faster. You will also be able to feel visible improvements in your overall health with the practice of intermittent fasting for a few days.

Intermittent fasting is especially more effective for women over 50 as it gives them a complete package. You can practice this simple lifestyle, and you will not only experience anti-aging and youthfulness but would also be able to lose weight rapidly. Your overall health would improve significantly and the risk of chronic illnesses would go down.

CHAPTER 8

IMPACT OF INTERMITTENT FASTING ON HEALTH

Intermittent fasting is a holistic health concept. It doesn't focus only on just one area of health like weight loss, blood sugar management, or hormonal balance but helps in balancing all and bringing them in sync.

As we have already discussed, most chronic health issues are a result of a gradual malfunction in several key areas. For instance, behind obesity, the reasons can be insulin resistance, excess calorie intake, poor blood sugar management, and hormonal imbalances. If you keep your focus only on managing just one problem, other conditions would keep working against your efforts.

Intermittent fasting helps you in balancing all these issues. You must understand that health is simply the absence of disease. When the systems in your body malfunction, you start feeling unhealthy. Intermittent fasting first helps your body in restoring the function of vital systems and then ensures that they keep functioning in sync and that's what makes it so effective.

Till now, we have discussed that intermittent fasting can help you in staying healthy and fit. We have also discussed that intermittent fasting can lead to weight loss, blood sugar management, blood pressure control, and other such things.

In this chapter, we will discuss how intermittent fasting affects our body and important health biomarkers.

Insulin Resistance

As you know, insulin resistance is one of the biggest health issues that most of us face but remain ignorant of. Insulin resistance is a condition in which your body stops responding to insulin signals, or the response becomes weak and slow.

This can cause the following issues:

1. Your cells would stop getting readily available glucose, and they will get energy-starved

2. Your blood sugar levels would remain considerably higher for longer than expected

3. Your body would face problems in glucose regulation

4. Your fat stores would increase as most of the energy consumed through food would start getting stored as fat

5. The insulin levels would remain very high all the time

6. The production of fat-burning hormones would be nil

The Cause

Insulin resistance can develop due to many reasons but the most common cause of insulin resistance in the body is poor eating habits. These days our eating patterns have changed considerably. We like to eat whenever we feel like. Having a few bites so very often have become a norm. Snacks have also become an integral part of our lives. All these habits lead to insulin resistance.

The Process

Whenever you consume food, the glucose released from the food invokes an insulin response. Every such incident leads to the release of a significant amount of glucose. Once released, the insulin can take anywhere between 8-12 hours before it dissipates completely. But, if you have a meal again after a few meals, it would again invoke another insulin response. This means that the overall level of insulin in your body would keep getting higher and higher as the day progresses.

Insulin plays a key role in facilitating the absorption of glucose into the cells. For this process, the receptors in the cells need to recognize the glucose signals. But, when the presence of insulin in the cells becomes perennial, the response of the insulin receptors goes down. They become resistant to insulin signals. This causes insulin resistance.

It takes years and sometimes decades for your body to fully develop insulin resistance. This problem is also very difficult to detect in normal blood tests as they are not looking for insulin sensitivity. The test to look for insulin sensitivity is HOMA IR. Another common test called HbA1c can give you a hint of the problem as it is used for detecting your blood sugar levels over a while.

Signs and Symptoms

Although you would need specific tests mentioned above to get an exact idea of your condition, yet the following signs can give you a clue whether you should take the test immediately or not.

Increasing Fat at the Belly: You are more likely to gain fat around your abdomen and not all over your body

The Feeling of Tiredness After Meals: Insulin resistance lowers the capacity of your body to process energy. The glucose absorption into the cells goes down, and the blood sugar needs to be brought down immediately. To make this happen, insulin starts the process of converting glucose directly into triglycerides. It is an energy-consuming process and it can make you feel tired.

Desire to Sleep After Lunch: This also happens because the body is not getting energy and has too much sugar in the blood. It simply wants some time to adjust the sugar and draw some energy. This is the reason you start feeling sleepy after lunch.

Inability to Lose Weight: Losing weight can become very difficult with insulin resistance as it is a fat-storage hormone, and as long as there is a high presence of insulin in the bloodstream, the process of burning stored fat wouldn't begin.

The Feeling of Fatigue on Waking Up: This is also a common complaint of people suffering from insulin resistance. Their bodies are struggling with the sugar management system, and that's a reason they don't feel rested even after waking up.

Extreme Thirst/Hunger: Thirst is a result of excess sugar in the blood that would generate a demand for more water. You may also start feeling more hungry because your cells stop getting the energy they require, and hence they keep creating a demand for food. You'd also feel cravings for sweets as they can provide that last drop of energy. This desire for sweets especially increases at the end of the meals because the body is unable to absorb the nutrients it requires.

Poor Concentration/Focus: Mind fog, lack of focus, and other such things are common with people suffering from insulin resistance as their mind also stops getting the glucose supply it needs to function properly.

The Solution

Intermittent fasting is one of the most reliable solutions for the problem. The main cause of insulin resistance in the body is the overexposure of insulin. It happens due to frequent intake of food. Intermittent fasting lifestyle helps you in putting a stop to it.

Generally, you can have anywhere between 2-3 meals a day within your eating window of 8-10 hours. This means that your system will get 14-16 hours period of zero insulin spikes. No new insulin spike incidents will occur in this period as you will not be consuming anything with caloric value.

As you know, the insulin present in your bloodstream starts to dissipate after 8 hours. The insulin levels will become extremely low after 12 hours. This means that your cells would have neither experienced any insulin calls for many hours, and now the insulin presence would also be nill. This gap helps the cells in developing sensitivity toward insulin.

Intermittent fasting is one of the best ways to reverse insulin resistance. The use of medicines like Metformin is common for the management of blood sugar levels, but it doesn't help in bringing down insulin resistance and have its side effects. From physical weakness to muscle pain, there can be a wide range of side effects. People also experience diarrhea, flatulence, abdominal pain, and low vitamin B levels while on Metformin. Intermittent fasting doesn't involve the intake of any kind of medication and hence it is safe from such side-effects.

Insulin resistance is just not a problem in itself, but as we have reiterated several times in the book, it is at the root of several other such illnesses, and hence by treating insulin resistance, you can ensure recovery from other illnesses too. From obesity to diabetes and high blood pressure to heart problems, most of the chronic health issues are somewhere connected with Insulin Resistance.

Fat Burning and Weight Loss

This is the topic women are most interested in, but if you look at a deeper level, weight loss is a natural process that would take place when your body gets healthy. You don't need to get healthy to get a toned body; you'll automatically get a toned body as you get healthy.

Fat burning and weight loss are some of the obvious effects of intermittent fasting. The process that's responsible for fat burning is Ketosis. As we had discussed, ketosis is the process of burning fat. It is the only process through which your body can burn fat.

The Cause of Fat Accumulation

Most people are unable to understand the cause of obesity and fat accumulation all their lives, and hence they keep struggling with the problem. Excessive calorie intake is just one part of the problem and doesn't tell the whole story at all.

The main cause of obesity in women is hormonal imbalance. This hormonal imbalance can be caused by several reasons.

- High levels of stress hormones called Cortisol in the body can slow down metabolism

- PCOS can lead to the release of several hormones that may cause obesity

- Imbalance in the thyroid hormones can also affect your metabolism and hence may lead to obesity

- Above all, insulin resistance is a major cause of obesity as it is also a common factor in all the issues mentioned above this

Insulin resistance works like a sledgehammer on your whole system and affects their functioning.

For instance, high cortisol levels or the stress hormone can slow down the way your body processes energy, but it is a fact that high insulin resistance can also be a cause of high cortisol in the first place.

When the insulin levels in the body increase and the blood sugar levels become unmanageable, the adrenal glands start releasing cortisol.

In PCOS, insulin resistance is at the bottom of most of the problems. Obesity, excess hair growth, male pattern baldness, high testosterone production, etc. are all the results of insulin resistance. However, in the case of PCOS, it is yet not known why it causes insulin resistance. But, one thing is very clear that you can manage most of the PCOS symptoms very successfully by reversing or controlling insulin resistance.

High insulin resistance is at the root of most problems, but one of its biggest consequences is fat accumulation.

- Due to high insulin resistance, the cells are unable to absorb glucose

- The blood glucose levels remain high as the glucose is not getting absorbed by the cells

- The pancreas senses the high blood sugar levels, and it pumps even more insulin to stabilize blood sugar levels

- More insulin means more insulin exposure to the cells, and it only leads to more insulin resistance

- When the cells are not absorbing glucose, the insulin needs to stabilize blood sugar levels by other means

- It first seeks to store the excess glucose as glycogen in the muscles and the liver

- The glycogen stores are not very big, and hence not a lot of glucose can be stored

- All the remaining glucose needs to be deposited as fat in the adipose tissues

- Insulin is the key storage hormone, and hence it signals the deposition of fat in the adipose tissues

A healthy person's body would be able to absorb most of the glucose as energy, and hence food would provide energy to the body. This is a reason you might have seen that kids seldom feel tired or lethargic after having meals. The food provides them energy. On the other hand, adults especially the ones in their late 40s and 50s, start feeling tired as soon as they eat anything. Their bodies are not able to process the glucose properly and that's why it happens so.

Due to insulin resistance, most of the food that you are eating is directly getting converted into fat. This is the reason they keep getting obese while their energy levels are at an all-time low.

Why Calorie Restriction Methods or Calorie-Deficit Diets Are Not the Solutions

Calorie-restriction or diets may look a lucrative and logical option; they don't offer a solution. We have already discussed that at the most, the calorie restriction can only offer the loss of water weight. When your body has high insulin resistance or due to your poor eating habits, the insulin levels in your body remain alarmingly high, your body is not in a condition to burn fat.

1. Insulin is the key fat-storing hormone, and hence in its presence, no fat burning can take place

2. Poor diet with high-carb intake means that your body is running on glucose fuel and hence it cannot start burning fat

3. The body reacts to the reduction in calorie intake by lowering the BMR and hence it also ineffective in burning fat

Therefore, most diets and calorie restriction methods ultimately lead to failures.

Wrong Results

One big misconception that people might develop when following a diet or calorie restriction program is that they may start feeling that their weight is going down. It is mostly a misconception.

This is correct that you would experience some drastic weight loss, but that is only the loss of water weight. The actual efficacy of the measure could only be observed through the reduction in the waist circumference. When your waist circumference starts to go down, you can believe that the weight loss measure is working in reality.

Here, you must also keep in mind that the fat releases more energy than glucose, and hence even if your body is burning fat, the reduction in fat would never be rapid. One gram fat releases more than twice the energy as compared to glucose. Hence, fat-burning would always be slow.

The best way to measure your success is to measure yourself on a scale and, at the same time, also put tape around your waist to ensure that the belly fat is going down.

The Solution

Intermittent fasting is one of the best ways to burn fat. It is a process that initiates the process of ketosis.

Ketosis: Ketosis is a very important process in which the body starts using fat as fuel. The fat is a very efficient fuel, and it produces more energy per gram. It is also a much cleaner fuel as burning fat produces fewer toxins.

Our body can burn both the fuel types. However, it likes to burn glucose as it is easy to use, and it produces energy instantly. But, that doesn't mean that glucose fuel is ideal. It is simply the fuel of choice due to its easy availability.

The fat fuel gives more energy and burns very slowly. This means that by burning even a small amount of fat, your body can sustain and feel energetic for much longer. It doesn't lead to a rapid decline in energy. If you feel that your energy levels go up and down rapidly, then also ketosis is the best solution for you.

Ketosis is a wonderful process. It can help in burning body fat, and it will make you feel more energetic and lively. However, there's one problem with ketosis that it can't happen as long as there is a high amount of glucose in your bloodstream. In that case, your body would automatically choose to go for the more convenient option and burn glucose.

Why Ketosis Take Place in Intermittent Fasting and Not on Diets?

When you are on diets, you lower your calorie intake, but you never really stop it. This means that after short intervals, you keep eating things in smaller quantities. This keeps causing insulin spikes and maintains a steady level of glucose in your bloodstream.

When you are following intermittent fasting, you stop taking meals for a minimum period of 14-16 hours, and this can go even longer. Our cells need energy after short intervals as they can't store energy and hence within a few hours, you start feeling the need to eat something. This urge is very feeble while you are asleep and that's why most fasting schedules are set for the night.

Once the cells don't get glucose, the insulin in your bloodstream metabolizes the glycogen stored in the liver for providing energy. However, these stores are very small. Fully replenished glycogen stores can last anywhere between 24-36 hours. This means that if you follow an intermittent fasting lifestyle, your glycogen stores would become weak within a few days, and then the next target would be the adipose tissues from where the fat would get metabolized for energy.

Why Is the Process of Burning Fat So Difficult?

The process of burning fat is very difficult, and it has been by design. The fat in your body is the contingency fund that your body saves for emergency periods of famines or crisis. Through its long evolutionary history, the body knows that there can be times when getting food can become impossible. In those conditions, only those would survive who can last on their stored fat for the longest. This is even more important in the case of women as they can also get pregnant in the meanwhile. This is the reason burning fat is so tough in the body.

If you want to burn fat, then ketosis is the only way to get results. There is no other way that the body can begin burning fat.

Now, there are several ways to initiate Ketosis,

- You can follow intermittent fasting, and that would lead to ketosis

- You can follow a keto diet, and that would also lead to ketosis. The results of the keto diet are even better with intermittent fasting

- Autophagy can also help in burning fat and initiating ketosis, but that's difficult. You can initiate autophagy better with intermittent fasting

Therefore, you can see that intermittent fasting is a great way to initiate ketosis and achieve faster fat burning.

Blood Pressure Regulation

High blood pressure is a problem affecting millions of women in the US. It is largely ignored because, in the beginning, it seems to be manageable. However, high blood pressure can be very harmful to various vital organs in the body.

The Cause

Poor salt-rich diet, high stress, and renal conditions can also be a cause of high blood pressure. But, one of the biggest causes of high blood pressure is insulin resistance and poor blood sugar management.

When your blood sugar levels are consistently high for longer periods, they can affect the density of blood and also the way other parts involved in the blood circulation function. Therefore, the management of blood sugar levels and insulin resistance is very important for lowering high blood pressure.

The Solution

Intermittent fasting helps in keeping the blood sugar levels low for considerably longer periods in a day. This is very helpful in keeping the blood pressure low. When your blood sugar levels are low, your blood would have to carry less water, and hence the lead on the kidneys would also go down.

Ignoring high blood pressure is a mistake many women make, but it can be a fatal mistake.

Poor Satiety Levels

This is the Achilles heels of most obese people struggling with their appetite control, especially women.

Numerous women feel extremely embarrassed about the fact that they are unable to control their hunger at the time of having food. No matter whether they have had a meal sometime back or not, they simply never feel satisfied with the food they are eating. There is no specific control that they know of.

This is a common problem that keeps making them feel embarrassed.

What most women don't realize is the fact that their inclination towards food can just be the result of chronic inflammation in the fat cells.

Chronic inflammation in fat cells is a common problem that can be caused by eating inflammatory foods, obesity, high oxidative stress caused by insulin resistance.

The body has a very organized system of indicating hunger and satiety.

When you are hungry, the gut releases a hormone called ghrelin. The function of this hormone is to signal the hypothalamus in the brain to indicate you to eat. This is the time you start feeling hungry. When you are hungry, the level of ghrelin secretion is the highest, as you eat, the level starts to decrease, and you start feeling less hungry.

Your fat cells store all the energy you are going to receive through the food you eat. They don't want to get overburdened. That's why even the fat cells have a mechanism to indicate satiety.

The fat cells also release a hormone called leptin. The function of this hormone is to indicate satiety. As you eat food, the level of leptin in your blood would increase as the fat stores would start getting filled up.

When you are hungry, the leptin levels are the lowest, as you eat, the leptin levels increase. High leptin levels indicate the hypothalamus that the fat stores are full, and you don't need to eat anymore and that's when the brain induces the feeling of satiety.

Here, it is important to understand that the leptin release would be proportional to the number of fat cells a person has. This means that a slim person would have a fewer number of fat cells, and hence the leptin release would be slow in such a person. The body would always want such a person to stock up a bit more. On the other hand, an obese person would have a higher number of fat cells and hence the leptin release would be much higher. This is the body's way of telling that the person doesn't need to eat more as there is a lot of fat already stored in the body.

This is a perfect system that is designed to prevent overheating and for the maintenance of health. Unfortunately, in the case of some obese people, this system malfunctions mostly due to chronic inflammation in the fat cells.

In their case, the fat cells in their body keep releasing leptin at moderate levels all the time. This means that even when they are not eating, and they are hungry, their fat cells are releasing leptin at a moderate level.

This should indicate the hypothalamus to stop you from eating. However, when the leptin release is constant at all times, and neither it goes down when you are hungry and nor increases when you are full, the hypothalamus gets resistant to the insulin signals and stops responding to it.

This means that even an obese person with chronic inflammation will have hunger as the ghrelin signals are working fine, but wouldn't feel satiety. The signal to trigger satiety stops working in them.

Poor eating habits and inflammatory food items play a big role in causing this problem.

Eating at frequent intervals and not paying attention to the things you eat can lead to this problem, and hence these habits need to be improved.

Chronic inflammation in the fat cells can contribute big time to obesity as it devoids the person of the feeling of satiety, and hence there is no real control over food intake.

Intermittent fasting can play a very big role in getting over this problem.

One of the prime causes of this problem is the habit of eating at frequent intervals. When a person eats at very short intervals, the brain starts getting overexposed to the leptin signals. It also puts a lot of pressure on the digestive system as well as the fat storage mechanism. The higher the amount of fat in the body, the greater would be the release of leptin.

Intermittent fasting plays a very important role in solving this issue. First of all, it helps in bringing down leptin exposure. When you start following intermittent fasting, your number of meals in a day goes down. They get limited to 2-3. This also means that there would be long periods when there would be no intake of food. These long gaps help in bringing down the automatic leptin release.

As the leptin release comes down, the hypothalamus starts becoming more sensitive to the leptin signals. You also start gaining better control over your appetite.

Here, it is important to keep in mind that chronic inflammation in the fat cells develops over a long period, and hence it can take even a longer period to get over the problem. You will have to show great restraint during this period.

- Your diet should comprise of anti-inflammatory foods that can help in getting over the issue

- Include more greens, herbs, and whole spices in your food as they have anti-inflammatory properties

- You must eat lots of things rich in anti-oxidants, flavonoids, and phytonutrients

- Include more things that have Omega 3 Essential Fatty Acids as an imbalance between Omega 3 and Omega 6 in the body is also a cause of the problem

- Reduce the number of times you eat in a day

- You must only eat till you start feeling 70-80% full because by this time you have eaten the required amount and leptin signals take a bit longer to signal complete satiety

- Eat mindfully

- You must not eat while talking to people or watching TV as the chances of overeating are high in such circumstances

These simple precautions can help you in getting over the satiety problem and may also help you in fighting several other chronic illnesses.

High Cholesterol and Heart Health

Heart health is a major health concern these days, and it is an especially big concern among the women over 50. Statistics show that every year hundreds of thousands of women die of heart problems in the US alone. Comorbidities like blood sugar management issues, diabetes, and high blood pressure increase the risk of heart problems several times over.

One of the biggest concerns in heart problems is the high cholesterol level. Commonly, cholesterol is taken as an umbrella term for fat deposits in the heart. However, that's not correct. Cholesterol is not the kind of devil it is projected to be.

Cholesterol plays a very important role in our body. It is the building block of the cell membrane. Even important hormones are made up of cholesterol. It also does the important repair work in the arteries.

Not all cholesterol in your body is bad.

- There is good cholesterol called HDL.

- There is Bad Cholesterol called LDL.

- Then there are triglycerides. They can be good or bad depending upon the kind of job they are put to.

Some people are so afraid of fat in the food that they are scared even to touch it with a ten feet pole. They fail to understand or are ignorant of the fact that dietary cholesterol has very little role to play in our body. Almost 80% of the cholesterol in the body is produced in the body itself.

The HDL or good cholesterol in the body is very helpful. The job of this cholesterol is to clear the blocking, and its level should be high in the body.

The LDL is the low-density lipoprotein or the bad cholesterol as it sticks to your arteries as plaque and blocks it.

The triglycerides are also the lipids that carry unused calories. In many cases, when you have insulin resistance and the insulin is unable to stabilize the blood sugar levels efficiently, it starts converting glucose directly into triglycerides to speed up the process.

High triglyceride levels are very bad news as it can be very harmful to your body. It can get deposited as plaque in your arteries; it can cause pancreatitis, blood sugar management issues, hypothyroidism, and many other such problems.

Blood sugar management is one of the most important things to lower your triglyceride levels. Losing weight, low sugar, and low carb diet, regular exercise, and a lower intake of trans fat (The worst kind of fat) can help you in lowering your triglyceride levels.

If the triglyceride levels go up very high, they can lead to the hardening of the arteries. This means that when there is some clogging of the arteries or when the arteries need to expand to pump more blood, they won't be able to do so and may result in a rupture. It increases the risk of strokes, heart attacks, and other coronary artery diseases (CAD).

Lowering your fat intake has neither any impact on your cholesterol levels nor on your heart. You need to lower the intake of bad fat like the trans fat or the things that may cause chronic inflammations.

Eating a lot of healthy fats can even help you in lowering your cholesterol level.

If you want to keep your heart very healthy, you must lower the intake of high-carb refined foods.

One of the best ways to improve your heart health and lower triglyceride levels is to follow intermittent fasting. It can help you in lowering the extent of insulin resistance, and that would, in turn, prevent the increase in triglyceride levels.

CHAPTER 9

INTERMITTENT FASTING- THE IDEAL LIFESTYLE CHANGE FOR WOMEN OVER 50

This is without a question that a reckless lifestyle is not going to take us anywhere. A lifestyle with no discipline and control would only lead to anarchy. If you don't have a fixed routine, getting up every morning even for a walk can become difficult. People even forget taking their medicines because they don't have a routine for it. Some restrictions are very liberating, and a fixed routine is one among them.

When it comes to health, you can get all kinds of health advice dime a dozen. If you add weight loss as a desired condition, then just the choice of options can be overwhelming. Fitness and wellness have emerged as a very big industry. You can get counseled for dozens of revolutionary procedures for weight loss that seem to work magically on paper and also on the models who never have been fat in the first place. This industry has been in place and thriving for the past few decades and has reached a market valuation of more than $70 billion. Yet. Somehow the obesity has tripled its extent in this world.

Even the weight loss industry, in the end, puts all the blame on the user for not following the process properly.

Not following a lifestyle is not a choice that you can afford. You can follow any kind of lifestyle, but having a healthy lifestyle would always be important.

One of the biggest problems with most lifestyle is that they are very limiting in nature and that's the reason most people are not able to follow them in the long-term.

The best thing about intermittent fasting is its sustainability. No matter your line of work or way of living, intermittent fasting can be followed by anyone.

It is a perfect fit for someone living in retirement while also being a perfect match for someone with a hectic traveling job. If you can't spare a lot of money for following a healthy lifestyle then also this lifestyle can be perfect for you or even if you keep your health above everything else, then too this lifestyle can be ideal for you.

It is one lifestyle that can work for you even if you shirk from exercise initially and would also work if you abhor dieting.

The flexibility in almost all the areas is the main forte of intermittent fasting.

Intermittent fasting is a very simple lifestyle with its focus on when to eat and not what to eat.

The importance of exercise, diet, sleep, and other important aspects of health don't become unwanted in intermittent fasting. They simply bring additional benefits to your results but your results would still come even if you just stick to the intermittent fasting lifestyle.

Intermittent fasting doesn't rely too much on other things to improve your health. It is a simple system to bring your vital functions in sync, and when these things fall into place, other things automatically start arranging themselves in order.

If you exercise, you would naturally lose weight faster, and your health would also improve rapidly. However, even in case you are not able to exercise, this doesn't mean that you will not experience weight loss.

The same is the case with diet. Intermittent fasting is a natural way to bring insulin sensitivity. This process helps in reversing several problems in the body. If you follow a healthy keto diet with intermittent fasting, your body would be able to get into ketosis faster. If you don't opt for a keto diet, the process of burning fat would get slow, but natural ketosis would still take place even with a healthy normal diet.

Intermittent fasting is a healthy lifestyle that helps in improving the natural processes of your body. Things like diet, exercise, better sleep routine, etc. will only help in improving the results.

It is a very simple lifestyle in which you only need to manage two distinct periods of feasting and fasting daily. This is an area in which there can be no major compromise. Everything else in intermittent fasting is adjustable, and we will discuss them in detail.

The ease of following intermittent fasting makes it so sustainable.

The reason for the failure of most weight loss methods or lifestyles is that they are difficult to follow in the long run. When you resolve to lose weight or improve your health, you feel very charged and pumped up for the next few days, weeks, and months. However, your resolve starts losing steam as you experience the hardships. The kind of temptation you feel for food on diets. The lethargy and fatigue people feel while doing intense exercises day after day.

Intermittent fasting puts you into so such constraints. The only condition in intermittent fasting is to maintain a fasting period of specified hours. Most of that time will be passed in sleep. Even when you are awake in the last few hours of your fasting window, you know that you will be able to eat after a few hours makes it easier to pass the time.

This is especially very important for women over 50 who are trying to adopt a healthy lifestyle as any strict routine will be very difficult to follow in the long run. There is a job, personal life, family, and several other things to balance at the same time and juggling all that with a strict routine can be very difficult and women most of the time choose to stick with their poor routine.

Intermittent fasting would come as a ray of hope in such conditions as you can manage it with any kind of lifestyle and responsibilities. You don't need to prepare extensive meals like in various diets; you don't even need to take out much more time for exercise as you can begin slowly and increase the tempo as you go along the way.

Intermittent fasting is a sustainable way to give your health another big chance and get healthier with minimum effort.

CHAPTER 10

HOW TO FOLLOW INTERMITTENT FASTING

Intermittent fasting is one of the easiest lifestyles to follow. It has immense health benefits. Most people believe that for a thing to work, it has to be complex and difficult. That is not the case with intermittent fasting.

Maintaining strict eating and fasting windows is at the core of intermittent fasting.

Let us discuss them in some detail.

Eating Window

First, let us begin with the easier part. This is the window in which you are allowed to eat.

This book is especially for women over 50, but let us first discuss women in general. Food is very important for the hormonal balance of women. Prolonged food deprivation can cause hormonal imbalance. This is the reason women in their reproductive age are advised against strict calorie-restrictive diets or even fasting for very long periods.

There are studies conducted on mice that demonstrate that longer food deprivation of any kind for a consistent period can cause shrinkage in the reproductive organs. It can also affect the hormonal secretion.

Therefore, young women should only practice only moderate intermittent fasting. Their fasts shouldn't be longer than 14 hours. They shouldn't even start with 14-hour fasts, to begin with. They should help their bodies adapt to the change slowly and gradually.

When it comes to women over 50, longer fasts can be performed without any restrictions as the risk of hormonal imbalances causing irregular periods or complications in conception and childbearing are not there.

Women over 50 have greater freedom in terms of the duration of fasts they want to undertake. This presents a very advantageous opportunity.

Women have a greater affinity to accumulate fat, but they are also more likely to shed the fat fast under the right conditions. Longer fasts help in beginning the process of ketosis and hence women can lose weight and burn fat much faster than men.

Hence, the hormonal conundrum that is a great problem for younger women doesn't pose much of a challenge to women over 50.

Women over 50 reaching their menopause get freedom from issues like menstruation. While this may be a great relief, other issues become more prominent.

For instance, problems like PCOS start troubling more where they should also have gone with their reproductive abilities. However, this doesn't happen.

Intermittent fasting with a correct diet can also help you in managing the symptoms of PCOS to a great extent. Frequent chills, mood swings, obesity, glucose tolerance issues, and other such problems wouldn't arise if you practice intermittent fasting.

Getting back to eating, women over 50 can take the liberty of holding longer fasts safely as they get more accustomed to fasting. They are at a lower risk of health issues arising due to hormonal imbalances caused by food deprivation.

Eating Hours in the Feasting Window

While women younger than 50 aren't advised to fast for longer than 14-16 hours if you have crossed your 50s, you can safely take it a notch higher to 18 or even 20 hours if you feel like.

However, in intermittent fasting, the number of calories you can eat holds very little importance, and the way and hours within which you eat them are way more important.

This means that your whole eating window, which spans from the time of the beginning of your fast until you finish the last meal of the day, is very important. This period is the eating window.

If you begin your breakfast at 7 in the morning and finish your last meal of the day by 5 in the evening, then you will have a 10-hour window.

Eating Discipline- Culling the Habit of Snacking

Another very important part of the eating window is following an eating discipline. You will have to improve the habit of eating.

We all eat mindlessly. We eat for the sake of eating. We don't mind having a few bites when invited to eat, although we may not be having any appetite or hunger. We feel it comfortably fine to have a glass of cold-drink when offered by someone even when we aren't hungry not realizing the fact that the glass of soft drink may have an equal number of calories as a full meal and to top it all; they are empty calories which are even more dangerous.

We get tempted to eat when an intoxicating aroma of food passes through our nostrils. Our desire to eat goes up when we see sweets and desserts on display.

We like to eat when we are sad as there are foods that provide great comfort. It is a sad fact that in the restaurants, there is a category of food categorized as comfort food.

We may only have two proper meals or less in a day but may have up to 10 incidents on average that may cause insulin spikes.

This is the habit of snacking that's causing the highest amount of damage to our system. Our digestive system gets crushed under a load of food, and it is unable to process that much food. This leads to the passing of most nutrients through the stool unabsorbed.

It also causes irreparable damage to our insulin system, causing insulin resistance. It overloads your whole pancreatic system making it overwork and the beta cells may lose the ability to produce the required amount of insulin in the future; this problem is known as diabetes.

The most important step towards following eating discipline is to stop eating indiscriminately. You will have to put an end to the habit of snacking. This is a habit that is only taking you towards a health doom.

You can only have 2-3 nutrient-dense meals in a day that can help in providing nutrition and energy.

To many women, this can sound intimidating, but it comes very naturally with practice.

You will have to begin by lowering the number of snacks you have in a day and then bring it to a minimum.

You will also have to eliminate sweets and refined carbs from your diet as they lead to food cravings. The more sweet you'll have in your diet, the faster you'll feel more inclined to eat. If you have more fat and protein in your diet, you'll feel less inclined to eat as our gut takes much longer to process them, and they keep releasing energy at a steady rate for much longer.

This is the basic preparation before you begin intermittent fasting. You must remember that intermittent fasting isn't some magical formula; it is a way to discipline the body to perform in an ideal way. This can't happen if you practice intermittent fasting but don't stop having snacks at short intervals in your eating windows. This would keep causing insulin spikes and your system would remain under duress.

Another thing with snacks is that they are mostly made up of refined flours and sweets. This makes them addictive, and you have stronger cravings for them. There aren't snacks rich in fat and protein as they would become proper meals then and you are less likely to feel inclined to eat after having them.

Therefore, eliminate snacks from your life, and you will be able to get benefits of intermittent fasting.

Fasting Window

Fasting windows are much simpler. There are very few restrictions in place apart from the eating ban. You can't eat in your fasting window is a comprehensive term, and it also includes consumption of calories even through drinking.

You are allowed to drink water, and it is very helpful to drink plenty of water as and when you feel thirsty. This will help your body in flushing out the toxins during the initial cleaning phase. But besides water, there are very few things that you can safely consume.

You can't drink any kind of sweetened beverage. You can't consume anything that has calories, even a few. This rules out all kinds of sweetened soft drinks, alcoholic beverages, fruits, and other such things. There needs to be a complete blanket ban on the consumption of calories in any form.

For women, in general, the fasting windows can range anywhere between 14-16 hours. However, if you are a woman over 50 and you have been practicing intermittent fasting for quite some time, you can experiment with longer fasts as long as you feel comfortable.

There is only one simple rule when you get accustomed to longer fasts, and that is not to overdo things. Try to maintain a routine.

Routine

It is a very important topic that seldom gets any limelight in weight loss, but it is equally important, like everything else. If you don't follow a routine, you'll find it increasingly difficult to follow a fasting schedule.

Have you ever noticed that some people eat very less or after very long intervals, and they don't feel hungry while you may find it hard to stay away from food even for short intervals?

This happens because our hunger system works like a clockwork.

As we have already discussed in the previous chapter that our gut releases the ghrelin hormone that creates the feeling of hunger. However, do you know that the release of this hormone works according to time and not as per your hunger requirements?

This means that if you are habitual of having your dinner at 8 in the evening, no matter what you are doing, you'll start feeling hungry by that time. Even if you had something to eat an hour earlier, you'd still feel the urge to eat at that time. This happens because the gut releases the ghrelin hormone on time and it creates the hunger pangs.

However, another interesting fact is that hunger pangs are temporary. This means that if you stop paying attention to these hunger pangs and divert your attention to something else, you may not feel the hunger pangs after some time. This happens because the ghrelin release is limited.

This is important to understand because shifting your fasting timings can have a toll on your tolerance.

For instance, if you start beginning your fasts around 6 in the evening and break your fasts as 10 in the morning, after a few days, your ghrelin release would get timed accordingly. This means that you'll start having strong hunger pangs in the morning at around 10 and around 6 in the evening to facilitate the intake of food. This would also mean that you will feel less inclined to eat during your fasting window.

However, if you follow an erratic fasting routine in which you begin your fast one day at 4 in the evening, 6 on another day and at 8 on yet another day, your ghrelin release would never be able to time itself, and you'll have to see longer periods of hunger pangs.

You will have frequent gastric juice release in your system when there is no food to digest and that can also cause problems like flatulence, and acid reflux.

Therefore, it is very important that you follow a fixed routine in your fasting schedule and don't change the timings very often. This will help you in practicing fasting in a much easier way.

CHAPTER 11

MAJOR DIFFERENCE IN VARIOUS INTERMITTENT FASTING PROTOCOLS

All intermittent fasting protocols are similar as they follow a standard format. You will have an eating window, and a fasting window in eat fasting protocol. The only difference among them would be the length of the fasting window.

This is very important to understand that the length of the fasting window is very important. The longer the fasting window, the greater the time your body would get for beginning the process of ketosis. The longer your body stays in ketosis, the faster would be the fat-burning.

This means that a 12:12 fasting protocol with an equal number of fasting and eating hours would have a lower impact on your insulin resistance, and the time taken for bringing your body into ketosis would also be much longer. However, it is only followed in the beginning stages.

The 14:10 fasting protocol is the most common protocol for women with 14 hours of fasting window. This fasting protocol gives you an ideal number of hours to begin ketosis. It also helps in reversing insulin resistance faster as the period of insulin absence increases in this protocol.

The 16:8 fasting protocol is generally most suitable for men as they get the greater benefit of ketosis, and hence they can burn more fat and gain muscles too. This fasting protocol is generally not advised to younger women in the beginning, as it can interfere with their hormonal cycle. However, they can build tolerance by increasing their fasting time bit by bit.

Then there is a 20:4 fasting protocol, also known as warrior fasting. It is a fasting protocol only suitable for women in performance sports or in areas where a greater tolerance is required. It is hard to practice and very strict to follow. There is no way that you can expect the 20 hours to pass uneventfully without giving you the hunger pangs. No matter how you time you fasts, you will get the hunger pangs anyway.

Some people also follow 24 hours fasts with fasting on alternate days. This fasting protocol also has its health benefits, but women should not follow these fasts as they can take a toll on your hormonal cycles.

The longer fasts are always more beneficial as they can help in beginning the process of autophagy. We will discuss this topic in detail in the coming chapters.

However, following longer fasts in routine can take a toll on the hormonal balance in the body of a woman, and therefore they must stay away from them.

Which Fast Should You Choose?

I have intentionally placed this chapter before the explanation of various intermittent fasting protocols so that your judgment doesn't get clouded. Most women feel attracted to the benefits of the longer fasting protocols, and they straight away pick the tougher ones. This is a fatal mistake that you must never make.

Fasting is a tough process. Through this process, you are putting your body under stress. Although the stress would be positive if it is exerted in a controlled manner, it can be too high if you don't have any control over it.

If you don't have the practice of keeping long fasts and you start keeping them, you are certain to experience hormonal imbalance. It would become very difficult for you to carry out your day to day activities, and all the benefits of intermittent fasting will be lost in the hormonal imbalance.

Women must never ignore the importance of observing fasts in a highly controlled manner.

If you want to observe longer fasts, you will have to build the capability from the lower levels.

You must begin by eliminating snacks and observing 12 hours fasts. When you start feeling comfortable with this routine for at least a fortnight, then only you should move to the 14:10 fasts.

You must stay at this level for at least a fortnight and observe the way your body responds to it. If you feel that you are comfortable with this schedule, then only you should move to the 16:8 and higher.

You must never try to jump the steps as this can not only be dangerous for you healthwise, but it can also affect your ability to make this process sustainable.

CHAPTER 12

VARIOUS INTERMITTENT FASTING PROTOCOLS FOR WOMEN OVER 50

We have discussed various intermittent fasting protocols briefly in the previous chapter, let us now elaborately discuss them.

12:12 Intermittent Fasting Protocol

This is the easiest intermittent fasting protocol, as it only involves fasting for 12 hours. However, you must not make the mistake of undervaluing these fasts.

When you begin these fasts, you will have to bring a sea change in your lifestyle, and for some women, this intermittent fasting protocol can prove to be the hardest.

When you have already started fasting for 14 hours, extending it for another 2 hours may not look like a very big deal. But, eliminating snacks that have been a part of your lifestyle for as long as you can remember can be a very difficult thing.

However, this is something that you must do.

In this fasting protocol, you will have to eliminate all your snacks. Your fasting window should begin with a nutrient-dense meal rich in fat and protein. This meal will help you in going from one meal to another without feeling the need to have snacks.

You will also have to keep in mind that just because you will not be able to eat for a few hours now, there is no need to overeat as fat and protein are calorie-dense, and they can provide you the energy to make it through the day.

You should begin your fasting window early in the evening around 7-8, as that will give your body more time to digest the food before you hit the bed.

This intermittent fasting protocol helps in conditioning your body for the long fasts, and it initiates you into intermittent fasting lifestyle.

The 14:10 Intermittent Fasting Protocol

This is the ideal intermittent fasting protocol for women. They get to eat for ten hours in this fasting protocol and then get a 14-hour fasting window.

The 14-hour fasting window is enough for promoting insulin sensitivity by causing insulin absence in the blood. It also gives your gut a greater relief from the abuse of food. It is also a time long enough to initiate the process of ketosis in the body.

The insulin levels in the blood begin to go down between 8-12 hours. If you have taken a balanced meal high in fats and low in carb, the insulin levels will go down much sooner. This would mean that the glucose in your blood would last much less, and your body will create energy demand soon. This would first lead to the depletion of the glycogen stores and then fat burning would take place with the help of ketosis.

Intermittent fasting is the easiest to follow because 14-hours of fasting pass very quickly.

If you are an early riser, then you must have your dinner early. If you want your day to begin by 9, you must finish your dinner by 6 in the evening. This would mean that your body would get at least 3-4 hours before hitting the bed. This much gap is sufficient for the proper digestion of the food. Even if you wake up around 5-6 in the morning, you will get at least 2 hours for doing high-intensity exercises, walking, swimming, or any other kind of physical exercise you want.

If you tend to stay awake till late at night, you can have the last meal of the day by 8. This would again give you a few hours before bedtime, and your body will be able to process the food better.

The toughest part of the intermittent fasting period begins around 4 in the morning as this is the time around which your body consumes all the glucose, and it is aggressively looking for energy. Your gut aggressively releases ghrelin to create hunger pangs. However, all that is useless because you are in your sleep. But, this is the time your body is releasing the fat-burning hormones most aggressively for fulfilling the energy demands.

Exercise in the morning would have a great impact on your overall weight loss story, and you'd find it extremely easy to lose a lot of weight even with a small amount of exercise.

This doesn't happen by magic.

The HGH Story

There is a hormone called the Human Growth Hormone in the body which has amazing fat-burning properties besides doing a hundred of other great things. This hormone assists in the overall formation of the body. From the soft tissues to the bones in the body, everything is made by this hormone. The production of this hormone is high in childhood, and it reaches its peak when you hit puberty. As you cross your teens, the production of this hormone slows down in the body. In adults, this hormone is produced in spurts. There are specific conditions in the body like hunger, absence of insulin and sleep that can help in increasing the production of this hormone.

Apart from its other benefits, HGH also has strong anti-aging properties that can help in reversing the signs of aging. It is also a very strong fat-burning hormone that can help in melting your belly fat faster. The best thing about this hormone is its ability to burn fat without causing the loss of muscle mass. It promotes the bulking of muscles while your muscle mass keeps on going down.

However, as you know, this hormone is produced by our body in very small quantities once we cross the teens. As we age, its production keeps going down.

Intermittent fasting can help in increasing the production of this hormone.

Intermittent fasting creates ideal conditions for the production of HGH:

1. It brings down the level of insulin, the most important condition for the production of HGH

2. It creates the energy demand which leads to hunger pangs

3. Mostly when all this is happening you are sleeping, and hence the production of this hormone is at its peak.

Studies have proven that intermittent fasting can increase the production of HGH by 1300% in women. This percentage can go as high as 2000% in men. Such a high percentage of HGH can give a great boost to your weight loss goals.

Therefore, when you fast for 14-hours, your body produces a lot of HGH, and it helps you in fighting obesity with greater ease.

When you wake up in the morning, the HGH levels in your blood would be very high. If you exercise even a little bit with high HGH levels, your fat-burning potential would increase tremendously. When you exercise with high levels of HGH in your blood, the HGH hormone will sense high energy demand and it would target the fat cells first.

In your eating window, you can eat 2-3 meals easily. This intermittent fasting protocol doesn't require cutting down your calories. You must not increase your calorie intake, but there is no need to reduce it further as this lifestyle can help you in bringing your weight down.

The 16:8 Intermittent Fasting Protocol

This intermittent fasting protocol is the most popular of all. The 14:10 protocol is also a derivation of this protocol for women as remaining in the fasted state for 16 hours may not be that helpful for some women in their reproductive age.

This intermittent fasting protocol is known for its ability to burn fat and build muscles. Due to this reason, this intermittent fasting protocol is also known as LeanGains.

The fasting period in this protocol is of 16 hours. This means that if you begin your fast around 6 in the evening, you will be able to break your fast at 10 in the morning the next day. You can adjust the beginning of the fasting window as per your morning routine. If you are a morning person, then keeping the fasting window early is always better, as hunger can become very aggressive in the morning.

The eight hours provisioned for eating are not suitable for three full meals. You can have two full meals and a very light meal in the middle.

This intermittent fasting protocol can give great results if you follow it properly.

The 16 hours of fasting in this protocol enable your body to burn more fat as there is an acute shortage of energy. If you manage your diet properly and don't consume too much carb-rich food, you can have amazing results.

However, you must remember that this intermittent fasting protocol has been designed primarily for men, and you must try this only after you have practiced 14:10 routine for some time. Practicing this intermittent fasting protocol directly can have side effects on your body.

The 20:4 Intermittent Fasting Protocol

This intermittent fasting is also known as warrior fasting, and it has a fasting window of 20 hours. As you can imagine, fasting for 20 hours can never be easy. No matter when you begin your fasting or how you time your fasts, you will have stretches where you will feel acute hunger.

This intermittent fasting protocol is not meant for normal people. This fasting style can help you in losing more fat much faster, but it also has a very strong risk of hormonal imbalance. One of the positive impacts of this intermittent fasting lifestyle is considered to be its ability to increase the production of HGH and testosterone. Now, as you may know, high testosterone production is good for performance enhancement. Hence, if you are in any kind of performance sport, this intermittent fasting lifestyle can help you, but it will also cause hormonal imbalance. High testosterone production will lead to lower female hormone production. It can also lead to hirsutism, male pattern baldness, hoarseness in voice, and masculine features. This is one of the most popular intermittent fasting protocols among the bodybuilder community.

This intermittent fasting protocol is not a new trend. It has been the oldest way of living our ancestors followed. During the hunting and gathering days, our ancestors didn't have a steady source of food. They needed to hunt in groups and could only afford to eat only once a day if they were lucky.

The warriors of the tribe went hunting at night and came back with the hunt in the morning. The whole tribe feasted on it and ate all they could. There was no means to store food, and hence eating everything was the norm. There was no fear of overeating.

This intermittent fasting protocol is also designed on the same principles. You need to fast for 20 hours. You get 4 hours to eat. There is no way you can have two full meals in a gap of 4 hours. It is always good to break your fast with some soup, then eat something semi-solid and then finally have something solid and nutrient-dense at the end of the fasting routine.

There is no need to watch the calories you are consuming. Because you only have one meal a day, you can eat as much as you can. This fasting protocol can give great results in terms of fat-burning, but it also has its side-effects, as mentioned above.

CHAPTER 13

AUTOPHAGY- THE KEYWORD IN HEALTH

Autophagy is a term that you might have heard these days. The concept of autophagy was in the study for some time, but no one was paying any real attention to it till recently. In the year 2016, a Japanese researcher Mr. Yoshinori Ohsumi got the Nobel Prize in medicine for his research on this concept and attracted the attention of the world.

The term autophagy means self-cleaning. The research has brought out that our body can clean itself of all the trash and toxins. It can do this without any outside help.

The study has highlighted the fact that our lifestyle has made the body very inefficient. We are living in an energy surplus mode, and hence the body becomes very complacent. It starts caring less about the useless processes going inside the body and these processes can cause a great deal of harm.

If the process of autophagy begins in your body, then your body can become like a printer or a machine that can clean itself or do self-repair.

Imagine that your body begins purging all the pathogens inside the body. This would include all the harmful bacteria, fungi, mold, viruses, parasites. All living inside your body thriving on the energy you consume through food. All such material would get cleaned in one swift sweep.

Your body will also develop the ability to process all the misfolded protein. When cells are produced in the body, many cells are not produced properly. They keep lying useless in the body. Through the process of autophagy, these misfolded proteins would get salvaged and would be used for producing energy and the raw material for new cells.

The process of autophagy can also bring an end to chronic inflammations as they are also using up the energy in the body. The process of autophagy can put to stop chronic inflammations.

Autophagy is designed to end all the processes in the body that are inefficient and energy-consuming.

It removes all the trash and toxins.

How Does It Begin?

Autophagy is the process that begins when your body is going through a severe energy crisis. It means when your body is not getting energy from any source. In that case, there is no other choice than to begin using fat stores. However, the process of autophagy is in place to ensure that only those processes are run on this energy, which is most essential so that survival can be ensured for the longest.

To initiate the process of autophagy, you must fast for at least 36 hours. This is the time taken for the body to exhaust the glycogen stores and the energy from glucose flowing in the bloodstream.

As soon as the body goes into an energy crisis mode, the process of autophagy begins, and it starts purging the unnecessary processes.

Once the energy from all sources is over, the fat stores begin to get utilized.

How Can You Initiate Autophagy?

The best way to initiate autophagy is to keep a long fast of 36 hours. Drink plenty of water during this period but do not eat anything.

However, if you want the process to begin early, follow an intermittent fasting lifestyle for a few days before keeping the long fast. Intermittent fasting also helps in exhausting your glycogen stores, and hence when you keep the long fast, you won't have to stay on it for very long.

Once the process of autophagy begins, you can also keep it running even by following an intermittent fasting lifestyle.

Autophagy is one of the best ways to keep your body healthy and free of all illnesses. It has been observed that the process of autophagy can be used for getting rid of chronic illnesses, infections, allergies, and other issues related to your immunity.

Intermittent fasting can help you in a big way to begin this process rapidly.

CHAPTER 14

INITIATING KETOSIS THROUGH DIET

If you want to lose weight and burn fat with the help of intermittent fasting, then initiating the process of ketosis should be your prime goal.

As you know, ketosis is the process in which your body starts to burn the body fat for energy. This is a very powerful process, and it gives out a lot of energy.

The fat is dense fuel and releases more calories per gram as compared to glucose.

However, as we have discussed, the process of ketosis cannot begin until your body is running on glucose. Therefore, there are only two scenarios in which your body would begin burning fat as a fuel.

Scenario 1: All glucose fuel gets exhausted

This can happen when you follow an intermittent fasting lifestyle. Intermittent fasting creates an energy deficit due to prolonged fasting hours, and hence glucose gets exhausted. However, this process can be slow as there is glucose in the bloodstream, then the glycogen stores are burned and afterward, some protein can also start metabolizing before the turn of fat comes.

Scenario 2: Your body is only getting fat to burn

In case you are only consuming a fat-rich diet, and the type of carbs consumed are complex carbs rich in fiber, your body will have a very limited supply of glucose. In that case, there would be no option than to burn fat from the beginning.

If you follow a high-fat, medium protein, low-carb diet along with an intermittent fasting lifestyle, the process of ketosis would keep running all the time in your body, and hence you will achieve greater fat loss as a much faster rate.

You must keep in mind that your meals should be nutrient-dense and must have the macronutrients in the given ratio:

Fat: This should form the biggest part of the meal. The fat percentage in your meal should be 70-75%. You must obtain fat from healthy sources. This means that although oil is a good source of fat, it might not be ideal. Instead, your fat must come from fish, meat, nuts, seeds, fruits like avocado, olives, etc. Deep-fried food items in hydrogenated vegetable oil can be very harmful as the good qualities of fat are over and it becomes very unhealthy.

Many people doubt that they may not be able to eat fat in such large quantities. They have no reason to worry as eating fat would make the quantity less. A gram of carbohydrate has 4 calories, whereas a gram of fat has 9 calories and hence you will have to consume less than half of carbs in weight to get the same number of calories.

Fat is processed very slow in your gut. This means that it will sit in your gut for hours before it is finally broken down by the bile juices. All this while it will keep your gut engaged, and hence the feeling of hunger or cravings will be less. Fat does not invoke a glucose response as it is broken down by the bile juices and hence it is very helpful in resolving the insulin resistance problem too.

Protein: This should be the second highest. At least 20-25% protein should be there in every meal. You can obtain goof quality protein from the lean mean, chicken, egg whites, legumes, pulses, etc.

You will have to be careful while having protein. It must always be taken in a very controlled manner. If you consume extra protein, then the body will start breaking the extra protein into glucose through a process known as glycogenesis. If you consume less protein, then your body will not get enough protein to make new muscles and carry out the required wear and tear as it isn't produced in the body. However, the body can't even store the excess protein for later use.

Whatever will be left will be converted to glucose. Therefore, you must be judicious in your use of protein.

The protein also takes the longest to get processed in your gut. It is more complex and takes much longer. This gives a unique advantage to you. If you have the right quantity of protein in your meal, you will not feel hungry very often as the protein will sit in your digestive system for long. It makes going from one meal to another without having snacks very easy.

Carbs: carbs should be the lowest in your meal. Only 5-10% of all the calories should come from carbs. You should only obtain carbs through whole grains and vegetables as they are complex and do not have very high calories.

The non-starchy leafy greens are the best to have as they have negligible calories and are full of fiber, antioxidants, flavonoids, phytonutrients, vitamins, and minerals. These vegetables will also take up a lot of space in your gut and keep it busy for long. The fiber in the leafy greens forms a gel-like substance that helps in cleaning the gut.

The whole grains are full of non-soluble fiber complex carbs. They also provide a lot of minerals, including the trace minerals that you can't get from anywhere else. The fiber in the whole grains is indigestible and it comes out in the exact form. It cleans the intestines properly and hence also prevents you from illnesses of several types.

You must avoid the consumption of refined carbs. They come from sources like sugar, refined flours, chips, bagels, crackers, processed food items, etc. They are bad because they lead to an instant release of energy into your bloodstream in the form of glucose. This will give you a good boost for the moment. But it will cause an insulin spike, and this energy is shortlived. This means that your body will start craving more energy very soon. This starts the process of frequent consumption of food.

Consuming empty calories is even worse as they provide a lot of calories but do not give anything to your system. Whenever you drink things like energy drinks, sweetened soft drinks, fruit juices, alcoholic beverages, sweets, and things laden with sugar, fructose, and maple syrup, they fill you with calories, but your digestive system won't get anything. However, as you consume anything, the digestive system prepares for the incoming load and releases a lot of gastric juices in anticipation. When it doesn't get anything to digest, these gastric juices affect the inner layer of your intestines and make them weak. The acid reflux experienced by you is also caused by this.

This is a reason you need to be very careful in the kinds of carbs you consume.

Following this diet can help you in losing your weight rapidly and getting healthier.

CHAPTER 15

BALANCING THE LIFESTYLE

Intermittent fasting is a significant lifestyle change. It may only look like extending fasting hours a bit or eating within specified limits, but internally a lot more is going on. When you follow intermittent fasting, your body starts its battle with excess fat, toxins, and chronic inflammations.

If you want to get great results from intermittent fasting, you will have to pay special attention to four important areas.

1. Food
2. Exercise
3. Sleep
4. Stress

Food: Food plays a very important role as far as our overall health is considered. Most people believe that exercise, gym, and other such things play a major role in their health. No doubt, these things do contribute to health but the biggest contribution is of the food you consume and the way you consume me.

The food you eat has an almost 85% contribution to your health. The rest of the things come in the remaining 15% percent. Therefore, you cannot underestimate the importance of food.

If you want to burn body fat, get rid of chronic illnesses, and have a healthy and fit body, then a good diet with intermittent fasting is very important. Ketosis is the process that can help you in burning the body fat, but as we have already discussed, if you keep having a high carb diet, it can become really difficult.

You must pay very close attention to your food and only have a healthy diet if you want fast and consistent results.

Exercise: In the previous point, we had discussed that food plays a very important role in your health. The role of exercise in good health also cannot be undermined. Exercise helps your body in developing stamina and immunity. Your ability to lose fat also increases when you exercise.

Intermittent fasting gives you a unique opportunity. When you follow intermittent fasting, the production of Human Growth Hormone and Adrenaline goes up. Both these hormones can help you in burning fat faster with very little muscle loss.

Studies have shown that intermittent fasting can boost the production of HGH by 1300% in women. This can give your fat-burning aspirations a great boost. Not only this, but a high HGH production is also good for more vitality and youthfulness.

If you can do High-Intensity Interval Training (HIIT) before breaking your fast in the morning, you can great results. HIIT is a great way to create serious energy demand in the body that can lead to fat burning. Doing HIIT on alternate days is a great way to stay healthy and fit.

In case you find yourself unable to do HIIT, you can still do mild activities like aerobics, dance or running. Even these exercises help in creating energy demand.

If you are unable to do even these, then going for walks in the morning and evening and swimming and other such activities must be carried out. These activities serve several purposes. They help you move a little, and that breaks the monotony and lethargy. Even some form of exercise also creates some positive stress in the body that leads to the release of chemicals like nitric oxide that helps in making your blood vessels more flexible. This can make a lot of difference in your health in general and heart health in particular.

Sleep: This is the third more important thing that you must never ignore. Most women, as they start reaching their 50s, find it increasingly difficult to sleep soundly. This may not look like a big deal in the beginning, but it can have far-reaching consequences.

Sleep disorders like sleep apnoea are common in women and they can have a big impact on your stress levels. When you are unable to sleep properly, the cortisol levels in your blood would go up and that can also become a reason for weight gain.

You will have to find ways to get a minimum of 7-8 hours of sound sleep. If you could sleep more then, it would be great but this should be least that you must have.

Most of the time, the reason for sleep deprivation is our overattachment with social media and electronic devices. You must try to make a routine and fix a time to sleep. An active lifestyle with some physical exercise in the day would also help you with sleeping.

Stress: We have already discussed the impact stress can have on your overall health. It isn't something that should be ignored at all. However, modern life has become such that stress has become a part of our lifestyle.

There can be no compromises when it comes to good health, and if you want to stay healthy, you will have to find ways to lower stress in your life. Try to find innovative ways to manage your time better and always make an effort to stay cheerful.

CHAPTER 16

MANAGING TRANSITION

Adopting a new lifestyle can be difficult. It is not much about the level of difficulty in the lifestyle but the changes. Every change in a lifestyle has some importance, and you will need to follow it. This is the point where most people fail.

The lifestyle we have been following has become a part of our nature. The difficulty you face in changing a lifestyle doesn't arise due to any technical difficulty but because you are habitual of certain things. This is something that you would need to change if you want to lead a healthy life.

The best thing about intermittent fasting is its sustainability. It is a lifestyle that will easily become a part of your life, and hence it is very sustainable. There are not many drastic changes that you may need to make and hence the transition is usually not very difficult.

However, you are bound to face problems if you try to bring drastic changes all of a sudden.

For instance, if you have been leading a life with no food discipline, following a 16-hour fasting routine, to begin with, can be very difficult. This is something that you must not do ever.

Proper Transition Is the Key

We have already discussed this point when describing the intermittent fasting routine. However, it is never enough to reiterate its importance, as this is the single biggest reason for failure.

Most women are in such a hurry of losing weight and getting slender that they want to begin with the toughest routine to get the fastest results, and this is where they fail.

If you want to get great results and maintain them for a longer period, you must mind the transition.

The best way to begin intermittent fasting:

- Starts by eliminating snacks

- Practice 12-hour fasts with only 3 meals in the eating window for as long as you get comfortable with the routine

- Move to the 14:10 fast and practice is for as long as you get used to it

- You don't need to start following 16:8 fasts as a ritual

- Keep following the 14:10 fasts but simply don't break your fast in the morning until you start feeling very hungry

- As you get into ketosis, you'll find it easier to go on without food as your body would be burning the body fat

- This will naturally help you in extending your fast timings

- If you are comfortable, then only extend your fasts to 16 hours or longer

- Never extend your fasts longer than 20 hours regularly

Autophagy is a great process, and you may want to initiate autophagy too. It has tremendous health results. However, it is a tough process and you must not fast for so long without practice. You should only keep longer fasts once your body has developed some understanding of fasting.

The longer fasts are good, but they shouldn't become a regular feature. You shouldn't practice them once in a few months. Practicing intermittent fasting regularly will also give you great health results.

CHAPTER 17

UNDERSTANDING AND MANAGING SIDE EFFECTS

Intermittent fasting is a major lifestyle change, and hence when you adopt it, your body may react adversely. This adverse reaction is usually temporary and just a sign that the body is adjusting to the new changes. You can also call these adverse reactions as side effects. The good thing is that most side effects that arise at the beginning of intermittent fasting are temporary and they would subside soon.

However, it is always better to know these side effects. There are some ways to even manage these side effects in a better way so that practicing intermittent fasting can become easier.

Some Common Side-Effects are:

Cravings

It is very common for you to have cravings. Either you go on a high-fat low carb diet, or you simply follow intermittent fasting, you will experience cravings in the beginning. These cravings are a result of energy demand created by the cells.

When you are living on a high carb diet, your body keeps getting glucose at short intervals. The cells absorb the glucose only for their immediate use and would look for energy very soon. When your diet comprises of refined carbs and sweets, your body gets an instant boost of energy. However, this energy doesn't last long as insulin needs to stabilize the blood sugar levels, and hence whatever is not absorbed by the cells is stored as fat. Therefore, when the cells again need energy, your body doesn't have any and hence you feel strong cravings.

When your diet comprises of fat, protein, and complex carbs, they release energy at a very slow and steady pace. This means that neither there is any sudden energy boost nor energy is absent. Your cells keep getting energy at a steady pace, and hence there are no cravings.

Your body will have to adapt to this change, and it can take some time. The best way to manage the problem of cravings is to eliminate refined flours, sweets, and empty calories from your diet. When you have a more stable diet, your body gets used to it and you would stop having cravings.

Headaches, Nausea, Lightheadedness

These problems are also connected with the issue explained above. When you adopt a fat-rich diet and follow long fasting periods, your body starts experiencing sugar withdrawal symptoms. Till now, it had been used to frequent insulin spikes and glucose boost. These instances provided energy to the body whenever it needed. However, it also leads to problems like insulin resistance.

Intermittent fasting and a fat-rich diet put an end to this cycle. Your body stops getting glucose boost at very short intervals, and that's why you may experience headaches, nausea, and lightheadedness. However, these problems are temporary and these signs would go away in a few days as your body adjusts.

If you want to relieve the headaches and nausea, you can have unsweetened black tea or coffee. Green tea and unsweetened fresh lime water can also help you.

Heartburns and Flatulence

These problems are caused by the changes in your eating schedule. As we have discussed, the ghrelin or hunger hormone release is timed in our body, and it also leads to the secretion of gastric juices. When these gastric juices can cause acid reflux issues that lead to heartburns. However, this problem will subside very soon as your body gets adjusted to your new eating schedule.

Here, the important thing would be to stick to the new schedule as a failure to do so can again result in heartburns.

Excessive Urination

You may find yourself in a position where you may need to make frequent trips to the washroom. This happens when your body is dumping the excess water initially.

This is a common thing and there is nothing to worry about. It would happen in most weight loss measures as your body tries to find a balance with the new energy routine.

However, it is important to note that your body doesn't just lose water, but it also loses minerals. You must replenish those minerals to stay at the top of your health.

The easiest way to do so is to mix a pinch of rock salt in water and drink it when you come back from the washroom. You will have to be careful here. If you have high blood pressure or any other issue related to your kidneys, this will not be an advisable thing to do. Drinking electrolytes is safer and better in that case.

You must keep in mind that dehydration can be a problem in the beginning, as you may rapidly lose water. This is a way for the body to get rid of the toxins. However, dehydration can cause a lot of health problems for you and hence that should be avoided.

But, you must also keep in mind that you should drink an excess of water as overhydration can also create problems.

A simple rule to follow is to drink plenty of fluids whenever you feel thirsty.

Intermittent fasting is a simple and effective way to stay healthy and fit. It is just not a weight-loss method but a way to achieve holistic health. These simple tips will help you in getting over the small obstacles that you may get on the way.

CONCLUSION

Thank you for making it through to the end of this book. Let's hope it was informative and able to provide you with all of the tools you need to achieve your goals, whatever they may be.

Aging is an unstoppable process, but it doesn't need to be difficult. With the help of intermittent fasting, women over 50 can make their life easy and stay away from chronic illnesses.

The risk of chronic illnesses starts increasing as we age. This is the time we need to become aware of the problems in front of us and work towards resolving them.

This book is an attempt to explain the ways you can work your way towards good health once you cross your 50s.

This book has tried to explain intermittent fasting for women over 50 in great detail so that you can get the full benefit of the process.

There is too much information scattered over the internet on all these issues, and most of it is contradictory. Through this book, I have tried to present all the facts in an organized manner so that you can sequentially understand them and take advantage of them.

In this book, I have tried to put all the facts in front of you. This book is not trying to upsell any concept to you or forcing you to follow a particular method. It has presented all the facts in front of you in an understandable manner so that you can be a better judge.

This book has explained the science behind intermittent fasting in a step-by-step manner and the ways it affects your health. It has also explained to you how you could get the maximum benefits of intermittent fasting.

I hope that you will be able to benefit from this book and lead a healthy and fulfilling life.

Finally, if you found this book useful in any way, a review on Amazon is always appreciated!